# of Health Care Governance

Redesigning Boards for a New Era

James E. Orlikoff
and Mary K. Totten

AHA books are published by American Hospital Publishing, Inc.,
an American Hospital Association company

This publication is designed to provide accurate and authoritative information in regard to the subject matter covered. It is sold with the understanding that neither the authors nor the publisher is engaged in rendering legal, accounting, or other professional service. If legal advice or other expert assistance is required, the services of a competent professional person should be sought.

The views expressed in this publication are strictly those of the authors and do not necessarily represent official positions of the American Hospital Association.

Library of Congress Cataloging-in-Publication Data

Orlikoff, James E.
   The future of health care governance : redesigning boards for a new era / James E. Orlikoff and Mary K. Totten.
     p.   cm.
   Includes bibliographical references.
   ISBN 1-55648-160-8
   1. Hospitals—Administration. 2. Hospital trustees.
3. Integrated delivery of health care. I. Totten, Mary K.
II. Title.
   [DNLM: 1. Governing Board—trends. 2. Hospital Administration—trends. 3. Delivery of Health Care, Integrated—trends. WX 150 O71f 1996]
RA971.O685 1996
362.1'068—dc20
DNLM/DLC
for Library of Congress   96-8523
                                                                             CIP

Catalog no. 196112

©1996 by American Hospital Publishing, Inc., an American Hospital Association company

All rights reserved. The reproduction or use of this book in any form or in any information storage or retrieval system is forbidden without the express written permission of the publisher.

Printed in the USA

AHA is a service mark of the American Hospital Association used under license by American Hospital Publishing, Inc.

Text set in Palatino

3.5M—6/96—0440

Richard Hill, Senior Editor
Lee Benaka, Editor
Peggy DuMais, Assistant Manager, Production
Marcia Bottoms, Books Division Director

James E. Orlikoff

> To my wife, Anita, because she is my partner.
> To my friend, Ahmed, because he asked me to.

Mary K. Totten

> To my family, who make my work worthwhile.

Contents

List of Figures and Tables vi

About the Authors vii

Chapter 1. The Changing Health Care System 1

Chapter 2. The Governance Transformation 9

Chapter 3. A Context for Governance in Systems 19

Chapter 4. A Framework for Effective Governance 39

Chapter 5. A Process for Restructuring Governance 61

Chapter 6. Issues in System Governance Structure 71

Chapter 7. Conclusion 89

Appendix. Case Examples of Governance in Integrated
          Delivery Systems 93

List of Figures and Tables

Figure 1-1. The Health Care Ecosystem 5

Table 2-1. Different Characteristics of Hospital and System Boards 14

Figure 3-1. Sample Compensation Committee Charter 34

Figure 4-1. Effective Governance Pyramid 41

Figure 4-2. Effective Governance Information Flow 52

Figure 4-3. Ineffective Governance Information Flow 54

Figure 4-4. Dysfunctional Governance Information Flow 54

Figure 4-5. Wesley Woods, Inc., Vision Alignment Matrix® (1995–1997) 58

Figure A-1. Henry Ford Health System Mission and Vision Statements 95

Figure A-2. Henry Ford Health System: Governance at a Glance 100

Figure A-3. Sharp HealthCare Mission Statement 101

Figure A-4. Sharp HealthCare: Governance at a Glance 106

Figure A-5. Borgess Health Alliance Mission, Vision, and Reorganization Goals 107

Figure A-6. Borgess Health Alliance: Governance at a Glance 111

About the Authors

James E. Orlikoff is president of Orlikoff and Associates, Chicago, a consulting firm specializing in health care leadership, organizational development, quality, and strategy. He is a nationally sought-after speaker and author on a variety of leadership issues.

Mary K. Totten is president of Totten and Associates, Oak Park, Illinois, a consulting firm devoted to publishing and education for leaders in health care and the arts. Ms. Totten has spoken widely, authored books and articles, and managed and evaluated grants on topics such as leadership orientation and development, service quality, mission stewardship, and strategic planning.

Chapter 1
The Changing Health Care System

The American health care system is experiencing revolutionary changes. These changes are creating new forms of health care delivery organizations and are forcing existing organizations to choose between an unprecedented type and pace of change or extinction. As the new forms of health care organizations emerge, new forms of governance will be required to lead them.

Changing Directions in Health Care

The reasons for the changes in the American health care system are many and varied and have been the recent fodder of front-page and network news: Forty million Americans (roughly one out of every seven) have no health insurance; the Medicare Trust Fund will face bankruptcy by the year 2002; the costs of health care continue to grow at a rate that exceeds the general inflation rate and, if unchecked, will reach 20 percent of the U.S. gross domestic product by the year 2000; the rising health care costs are inhibiting the ability of American businesses to compete in a global economy; the payers of health care are becoming more sophisticated and demanding; and on and on.[1] Paradoxically, as more money is spent on health care, the argument can be made that the health status of the population is actually declining due to increases in tuberculosis, AIDS, violence, infant mortality, and so on.

As a result of these and other pressures, market and governmental forces are reshaping the health care landscape dramatically. Consequently, the health care environment and the health care organizations within it will be remarkably different. Following are descriptions of current trends that are gaining steam.

Although all players in the health care market are being affected by the changes, two groups in particular are experiencing unprecedented pressure: independent, freestanding acute care hospitals; and solo or small group practice physicians. Hospitals and physicians together account for almost 60 percent of all health care spending and thus are the targets of massive reductions in reimbursement.[2] There will be a massive reduction in hospital capacity via mergers, closures, integrated delivery system (IDS) formation, and downsizing. In addition, there will be a corresponding reduction in physician capacity, as some predict a surplus of 150,000 physicians by the year 2000.[3]

The way that care has been delivered in the past is too expensive to maintain and will change in the future. Reductions in Medicare and Medicaid payments to providers and the actions of other aggressive and informed payers are seeing to that. Specifically, providing care in an inpatient, acute care hospital setting, with an emphasis on specialty-focused, fragmented care no longer will be the norm. Rather, necessary cost efficiencies will be obtained only by the transition to a continuum of outpatient services with a primary care focus and by the minimal use of inpatient services.

Accelerating this trend is the decline of fee-for-service health care and the rise of managed care. Aggressive payers are realizing that the best way to control the growth in health care costs is to *make the providers of care assume the financial risk for the care.* Thus, the trend of at-risk capitation is growing fast. Under this system, a hospital or other provider is either a member or an owner of a managed care network that collects a set amount of money or premium from a payer for each person or "head" (capitation) to provide all health care for a set period of time. If the network can provide care costing less than the premium collected, it makes money; if it provides care costing more than the premium collected, it loses money. Here, the provider is at risk and hence has the greatest incentive to control costs.

These reversed financial incentives are resulting in radical changes in hospitals as they move from being freestanding revenue-generating centers to cost centers that are part of integrated health care delivery networks. The independent, freestanding acute care hospital will be hard-pressed to survive when it becomes impossible to make money treating inpatients and when outpatient care can be provided less expensively by integrated networks.

Additionally, the focus of health care delivery is shifting from predominately providing services to people who are ill or injured to providing services to communities that are designed to keep people well (preventing or minimizing illness or injury). Because of this, and because of the changing financial incentives, in the near future, health care providers may be offering a variety of services that today fall into the category of "alternative medicine." The term *alternative medicine* describes therapies that are outside conventional medical and surgical norms and are not usually taught in U.S. medical schools.[4] Many of these alternative treatments rely on behavioral changes to improve health status, and avoid invasive procedures. Thus, they do not require an acute care inpatient or high-tech outpatient setting and are likely to be much less expensive than traditional medical treatments.

Other trends include the changing focus on quality. Quality now is emerging as a strategic competitive imperative, with health care organizations and networks competing to attract and retain payers on the basis of the objectively demonstrable high-quality, cost-efficient care they are providing. Efficient markets operate on information, and as the health care market becomes more efficient, it demands more information from health care providers regarding quality as well as costs. Health care providers may compete on the basis of cost, but they will differentiate on the basis of quality.

Thus, the health care environment is being reformed by forces such as informed and aggressive payers and employers, the growth of managed care and at-risk capitation, the increasing availability of quality data, reductions in Medicare payments, the linking of health care financing and delivery systems, the movement away from inpatient acute care, the increasing emphasis on wellness and illness prevention, the growth and acceptance of alternative medicine, and many more. Individually, any of these changes is significant; together, they are revolutionary. Effective leaders of health care organizations realize that these changes are not in the distant future but, rather, are happening now, and therefore these effective health care leaders are acting now.

The New Health Care Ecosystem: The Integration Imperative

Both government and private purchasers of health care are demanding value (high quality at low cost) for their health care dollar. This is creating irresistible pressure on hospitals to change the way health care is organized and delivered. To provide the value that the market demands, hospitals and health care systems must integrate all of their many and diverse clinical and operational functions. This includes integration of physicians, clinical services, information systems, inpatient and outpatient access points, governance, quality improvement, and all parts of the health care continuum.

As a result of these pressures and trends, a new ecosystem is emerging in health care. An *ecosystem* is simply a system formed by the interaction of a community of organisms within their environment. A forest ecosystem, for example, may be used as an analogy for the emerging health care ecosystem. In the forest, the source of all life is the sun. The organisms in the forest have a simple goal: to position themselves to absorb as many of the rays of the sun as possible. If they are unable to do this, they must try to eke out an existence as a niche player, evolving mechanisms to survive on diminished sunlight.

Those organisms attempting to maximize their exposure to the sun try to grow as tall and broad as possible. By this strategy, the trees also attempt to *block the rays of sun from their competitors,* causing their competitors to whither and die.

Drawing on this oversimplified example of the forest ecosystem as an analogy for the health care ecosystem, figure 1-1 shows that the source of life in the health care ecosystem are the payers of care. These are not the insurers of health care but, rather, the purchasers of health care — the government, employers, and large businesses, for example, that actually pay the costs of health care.

The major challenge to the organisms in the health care environment is to get as close as possible to the payers. Just as the tree attempts to maximize its exposure to the sun, the provider of health care must try to get as close as possible to the purchaser of health care. This relationship requires that the health care provider assume the risk, but in exchange for assuming that risk, the provider controls the majority of the premium dollar, gains access to the majority of the covered lives or enrollees, and thus has the best chance to control its own destiny.

The farther from the source of life a provider is in the health care ecosystem, the less likely the provider is to survive. The types of organisms in the health care ecosystem that are best prepared to thrive and that offer the most effective competition to niche players are IDSs. As figure 1-1 shows, those providers having the least degree of integration occupy the least desirable positions in the health care ecosystem. For example, independent physicians and freestanding acute care hospitals are at the bottom of the health care ecosystem's food chain.

The Integrated Delivery System

As health resources become more scarce and tightly controlled, hospitals will have to integrate their services with those of other health care providers to use those resources more efficiently. The forces of the market in its demand for efficiency as the new ecosystem emerges push health care providers to create, evolve into, or affiliate with IDSs.

Gillies and colleagues define *integration* as "the extent to which functions and activities are appropriately coordinated across operating units . . . so as to maximize the value of services delivered."[5] The promises of integration are clear: better service to the community, greater continuity of care, greater control over quality and costs, and increased efficiency, to name a few.

Figure 1-1. The Health Care Ecosystem

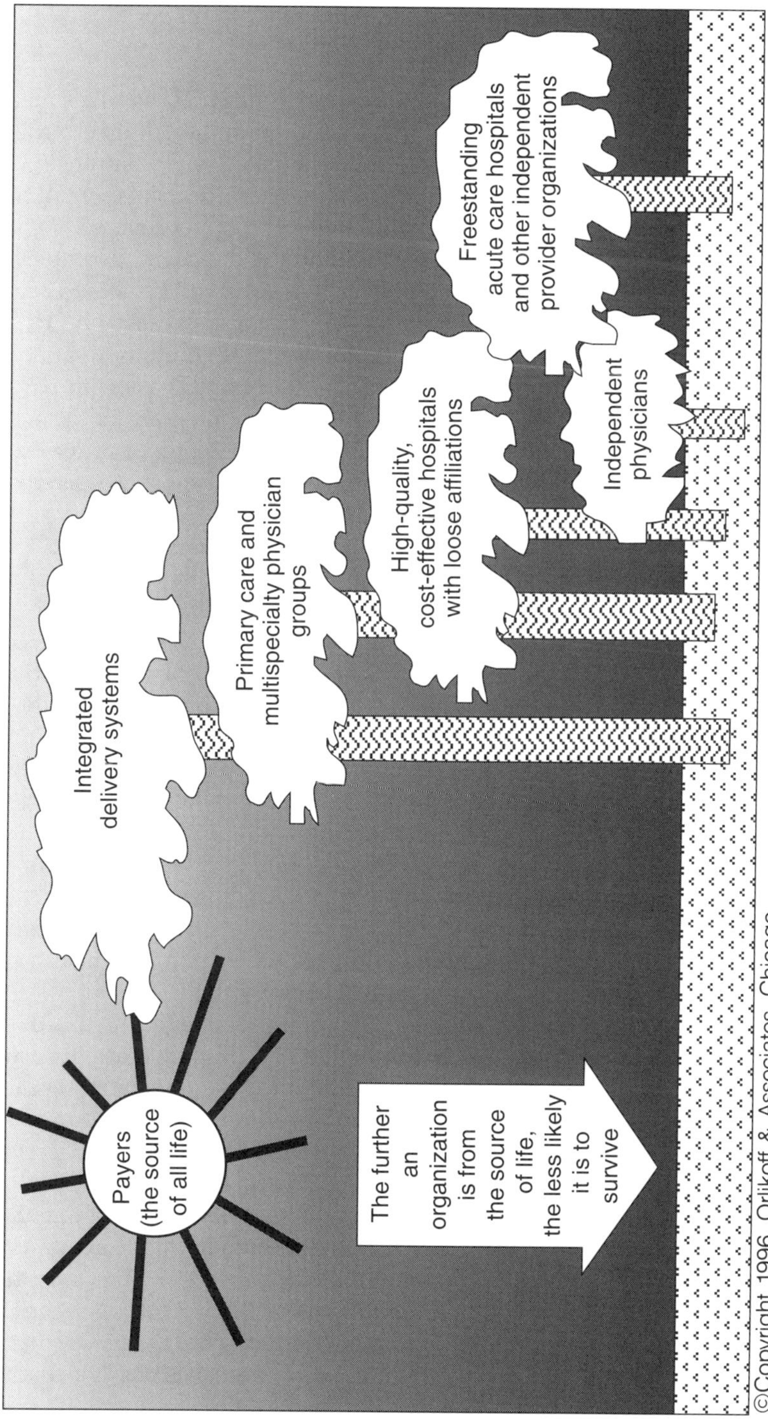

Integrated delivery systems

Primary care and multispecialty physician groups

High-quality, cost-effective hospitals with loose affiliations

Freestanding acute care hospitals and other independent provider organizations

Independent physicians

Payers (the source of all life)

The further an organization is from the source of life, the less likely it is to survive

©Copyright 1996, Orlikoff & Associates, Chicago.

An IDS has the following characteristics:

- *It integrates the delivery of care with the financing of care.* This means that the organization not only will provide health care but also will perform functions heretofore associated with insurance companies, such as the actuarial assessment and management of risk, the calculation and monitoring of claims cost per covered life, and the negotiation and execution of contracts directly with employers and other purchasers of care. Further, IDSs will be able to accept a variety of payments, ranging from full at-risk capitation to fee-for-service. Also, IDS services are available through a variety of innovative financing arrangements and partnerships with payers. Although not all health care systems have integrated a financing piece (such as a health maintenance organization or other insurance function), the leading systems have and most other systems are currently trying to do so.
- *It integrates physicians with the organization.* A core principle of business economics is that the fundamental means of production must be controlled by a business. Physicians are the fundamental means of a health care organization's production and so must be controlled by the organization. How this control is most effectively achieved (physician as owner, partner, employee, stakeholder) is still a matter of debate. But to be truly integrated, the IDS must share risk and align incentives with its physicians. Further, integration with physicians must maintain a proper balance between primary care physicians and specialists.
- *It provides a highly accessible continuum of care.* This continuum of care and services is based on decentralized primary care provider locations, and smooth and efficient access to specialty care, hospital care, and ancillary services. Multiple access points to health care across this continuum is a key characteristic.
- *It assumes accountability.* The IDS is accountable for the health status of specific populations in defined geographic areas. Its activities can be more focused and effective than a hospital's because they (1) are based on the identified needs of specific communities and populations and (2) include promoting health and prevention, not just treating injury and illness. The IDS is available to the entire community and is committed to the health of the entire community, not just its enrollees or covered lives. Pointer and colleagues state that accountability "may prove to be the most fundamental distinguishing characteristic of" IDSs.[6] Although the idea of complete community accountability is accepted as a goal of mature IDSs, few have truly reached this point as yet. It is possible that this

will not be attained until both an IDS and the market within which it exists are mature.
- *It provides high-quality, cost-effective care due to its integration of different individuals and entities that provide similar levels of care.* It also achieves economies of scale because of its size, and conducts effective training and information sharing programs for its providers.
- *It has and relies on an effective, unified cost and quality information system.* This is essential to the integration of patient care and to the ability to monitor and control quality and cost efficiency. As a result of this information system, IDS leaders are able to quickly determine the true costs and quality of any of their discrete services or procedures.
- *It integrates physicians at all levels of its leadership structures and planning activities.* Clinical leadership is key to IDS success.
- *It is led by a new form of integrated, systems-oriented governance.*

Implications for Health Care Governance

Whether or not the IDS emerges as the dominant organism or as a transitional form to some other type of organism that will occupy the top of the food chain, massive changes are ahead for hospitals, multihospital systems, and all health care providers. Hospitals will not be able to survive unchanged, nor will traditional hospital governance or newer forms of health care organization governance.

All the changes in health care—the emerging ecosystem; the ascendance of IDSs; the consolidation of health care providers via mergers, closures, and integration—will require new forms of governance. As new forms of health care organizations emerge, new forms of governance will be required to lead them. Currently, there is a tremendous degree of variance in governance sophistication. Although many boards have gone through some form of transition, a quantum leap to the next new form of governance is required.

Why will new forms of governance be required? To oversee and manage the incredibly complex and interdependent relationships that form the complicated organisms that are integrated delivery systems. These relationships (with the physicians, the senior managers, the community, the purchasers, the multiple institutions and boards, to name a few) are as critical to the success of the system as they are complex and transitory, and they must be nurtured effectively.

To assist boards and their members in the challenging task of transforming themselves, this book examines the forms and functions of changing governance in changing times and presents conceptual and practical models of effective governance function and structures.

References

1. Orlikoff, J. E., and Totten, M. K. An action plan for boards: leading your organization into health reform. *Health Governance Digest* 3(5): 1–6, Sept.–Oct. 1993.
2. *AHA News* 30(48):3, Dec. 5, 1994.
3. Pew Health Professions Commission. *Shifting the Supply of Our Health Care Workforce.* San Francisco: University of California, 1995.
4. Eisenberg, D. M., Kessler, R. C., Foster, C., and others. Unconventional medicine in the United States: prevalence, costs, and patterns of use. *New England Journal of Medicine* 328(4):246–52, Jan. 28, 1993.
5. Gillies, R. R., Shortell, S. M., Anderson, D. A., Mitchell, J. B., and Morgan, K. L. Conceptualizing and measuring integration: findings from the health systems integration study. *Hospital and Health Services Administration* 38(4):467–89, Fall 1993.
6. Pointer, D. D., Alexander, J. A., and Zuckerman, H. S. The governance challenge: preserving community mission with integrated health care systems. *Frontiers of Health Services Management* 11(3):6, Spring 1995.

Chapter 2
The Governance Transformation

As the health care environment and the character and function of health care organizations change, so too will governance change and evolve. The not-necessarily-linear transitions from hospitals to multihospital systems to integrated delivery systems (IDSs) to health care systems that truly accept the mantle of accountability for the health of their communities all will involve different forms of governance. For example, governance of an IDS may be very different from governance of a hospital (governance of a facility is very different from governance of an organization responsible for the health of a community). Yet one of the constants of governance is the ultimate accountability of the board to the mission of the organization or system it governs.

The Evolution of Governance

Governance of health care organizations is undergoing many rapid transitions. Among the more significant governance transitions are:

- *The transition from governance focused on local communities and constituencies to a more regional focus with more disparate constituencies:* As hospitals merge and form IDSs, the system board finds itself with a broader constituency than that of the hospital board. This is due to the system's expanded geographical coverage and to a new emphasis on the health of the entire community, not simply a segment of it that avails itself of the health care organization's services.
- *The transition from market share defined as admissions and inpatient census to market share defined as covered lives and physicians:* With the rapid rise of managed care and capitation, standard measures of capacity (such as number of hospital beds) and demand (such as admissions and census) become obsolete and yield to new

measures. The new measures of health care organization or IDS capacity include the number of aligned physicians and the proper balance between primary care and specialty physicians. New measures of demand include the number of covered lives served by the organization or system, as well as the size of the communities for which the system accepts accountability for health. Boards in this environment must transition to, and become adept at, maneuvering new levers of control to balance capacity and demand. This is a critical transition for governance because managed care reduces costs in a system by more than simply reducing inpatient days and eliminating unnecessary treatment. It forces the reduction of health care capacity, such as decreases in the number of hospitals, hospital beds, or specialist physicians in a particular market.

- *The transition from cost-based pricing to price-based costing:* In inefficient markets, the way the provider of a good or service develops the price for that good or service is based on its cost. By simply adding a margin on top of the cost, the price is determined. However, as markets become more efficient, cost-based pricing loses currency as the market demands lower prices. When the market is efficient, the market does not "care" what the cost of a good or service is, only what the lowest price is. At this point, cost-based pricing yields to price-based costing. Under this method, the provider of a good or service determines what the market is willing to pay for the commodity and then reengineers the process to produce the good or service at a cost that is below market price. A classic example of this dynamic is the transition of fee-for-service health care to capitation. Boards must change their focus to cope with, and preferably lead, this transition by ensuring that (1) the costs of the services provided by their system are known, (2) they are appropriate relative to the capitated rate, and (3) constant organizational efforts to lower costs are under way.

- *The transition from managing stability to leading change:* In stable times, the role of the board was to be reactive, to monitor the past. In times of turmoil and massive change, the fundamental role of the board becomes one of creating the future through forward-thinking, proactive planning and action. This requires boards to move away from a cumbersome, slow decision-making process to a streamlined, rapid one.

- *The transition from institutional (local) board authority to system (central) board authority:* As IDSs form through mergers and affiliations of hospitals and other health care providers, many boards that previously had ultimate authority for their organizations now find that they are subordinate to a system board. The reconciliation of this diminution of authority along with the clarification

of relative roles and authorities between the subordinate and system board are crucial to effective system governance.
- *The transition from representational governance to systems-thinking, mission-driven governance:* Many hospital and health care organization boards are composed of members who were explicitly or implicitly chosen (or who believe it is their role) to "represent" specific constituencies or organizations. This gives rise to representational governance, where the members of the system board do not focus on the best interests of the system as a whole but, rather, focus on the best interests of component parts of the system. Representational governance is the antithesis of integration. An IDS should have integrated, mission-based governance.

  The way to overcome representational governance is not through an emphasis on structure, such as how board members are chosen, or whether there are few or many boards. For example, board members selected from the representative components of the system will not necessarily function as a representative board if they have a mission focus and are trained in systems thinking, as discussed in chapter 3. The issue is not how board members are selected but, rather, how they are trained and focused. Structure (such as centralized or decentralized governance, board member selection processes, or multiple layers of governance discussed in chapter 6) alone does not prohibit representational governance. The way to overcome representational governance is through a mission focus and an emphasis on systems thinking in governance.

  Systems thinking means that the board members of local institutions recognize that the interests of their institutions, communities, or constituents will be best served in the long run if the system as a whole pursues and achieves its mission. It also means that members of a system board place the best interests of the system above those of the constituency or institution from which they came. As IDSs form new alliances that are not based on ownership but on a commitment to shared objectives, systems thinking becomes even more critical to successful integration and effective system governance.
- *The transition from the governance of facilities to the governance of services:* As IDSs and hospitals push patient care outside the boundaries of the acute care environment, and as they increasingly focus on providing preventive and wellness services to a broader community, the context of health care delivery changes and transcends the building or institution. Thus, governance of IDSs moves away from governance based on institutions and toward governance based on services. This presents a challenge because it is easier to govern a building such as a hospital—and what goes on inside

it—than it is to govern a disparate collection of services provided in a widely dispersed manner and geographic area.
- *The transition from a focus on the individual via acute care and care of illness to a focus on the group or community via a continuum of care and prevention of illness:* There is a law of economics called the Fallacy of Composition that states that what is good for the individual is not good for the group and, conversely, what is good for the group is not good for the individual. Until recently, health care has focused on the sick individual, with the result being a diversion of resources away from community health and a resulting decline in the health status of the population.

With the growth of managed care and capitation, financial incentives for health care providers are shifting away from sickness care and toward prevention, wellness, and health maintenance. Under managed care and capitation, the incentive for a health care organization to provide services to keep its enrolled population or covered lives healthy is clear. But why should the board of a health care organization be concerned with the health status of its entire community, including those who are not enrolled in its health plans or among its covered lives?

Effective health care leaders realize that the overall community will inexorably influence the health of the organization's enrollees or covered lives. Therefore, the health care organization must become intimately involved in and accountable for assessing and maximizing the health of the entire community. Health systems today are looking far beyond disease prevention and wellness to issues such as crime and poverty and their impact on overall community health. To be effective, health care organization leaders will have to measure their organization's impact on community health and use the outcomes to maximize leverage in improving the health status of the community.

Community health improvement initiatives are effective investments in positioning for the future of managed care and fixed-premium health care delivery. Perhaps more important, they are consistent with the missions of health care organizations and reflect an ethical commitment critical to the future of health care delivery.

However, the downside of this is that boards will have to balance the needs of the group against those of the individual. Managed care involves population-based health care, which means that more emphasis is placed on the group and community health than on the individual and sickness care. To make this rhetoric a reality, boards will increasingly need to realize that as more of their organization's resources are devoted to the community, fewer will be available to provide services to sick individuals. This means

that rationing of care for individuals so that services can be provided to the community will be an issue that all IDS and hospital boards will have to address in the near future.
- *The transition from simply delivering care to delivering and financing care:* As mentioned in chapter 1, one characteristic of an IDS is that it not only provides health care, but also performs functions relating to the financing of care. These functions include the acceptance and processing of premium dollars; actuarial assessment and management of risk; the calculation and monitoring of medical loss ratios (how much of the premium dollar is actually devoted to health care); and many others.

  This means that IDS boards will need to merge a focus on health care delivery (such as that of a hospital board) with a focus on health care financing (such as that of an insurance company board). This will entail new skills, new structures, and new challenges for governance.
- *The transition from governance oversight of physicians to physician involvement in governance and leadership of the system:* For an IDS to be successful, physicians must be integrated into all aspects of the system, including its board(s) and other leadership structures. Boards will need to reconceptualize their relationships with physicians, which at a minimum will necessitate greater physician involvement in governance.

The preceding transitions in governance can be seen as leadership paradigm shifts from governing hospitals to governing systems.

As research results confirm, health care organization governance is changing in response to an industry in transition. Research conducted by The Governance Institute on the boards of 50 not-for-profit hospitals and 65 not-for-profit health systems reveals emerging differences between hospital boards and health system boards.[1,2] According to the studies, governance differences are evident in that system boards are smaller, meet less frequently, compensate their members more often, and spend more time on formal education than do hospital boards. Specific differences can be seen in table 2-1, which is drawn from the two Governance Institute studies.

The New Imperative to Create the Future

Health care currently is confronting what futurists call "the two-curve problem." Basically, the two-curve problem relates to:

> . . . a business or industry that is on a stable . . . curve confronts a second curve—"a new world order"—that transforms the existing

Table 2-1. Different Characteristics of Hospital and System Boards

Characteristics of Sample	Hospital Boards	System Boards
Average size	18 members	13 members
Range in board size	5–45 members	6–51 members
Percent that offer cash compensation to their board members	4%	14%
Percent that impose term limits for board members	78%	70%
CEO is a member of the board	77%	76%
Average amount of time devoted to formal board education per year	16 hours	23 hours
Percent that meet:		
Monthly	74%	44%
Bimonthly	18%	29%
Quarterly	8%	27%
Average number of standing committees of the board	6	5
Percent with the following committee:		
Finance	93%	78%
Executive	79%	75%
Planning/strategy	79%	56%
Nominating	46%	53%
Compensation	31%	48%
Quality improvement	65%	28%
Percent that have a line item in budget for governance (education, development, and so forth)	28%	26%
Average number of nonboard members who attend board meetings	8	6

business or industry and threatens to replace or surpass the original curve. . . . The two-curve problem presents difficult choices for [leaders] because the pace of change is uncertain and the degree to which the second curve will surpass the first is unclear. Compounding the dilemma, the first curve is usually very profitable and the second curve very risky.[3]

In health care, the old, profitable curve is based on fee-for-service payment for acute illness care, with the hospital as a major player in the system. The second curve is based on capitated payment (or severely discounted fee-for-service payment) for primary care in a community setting, with the IDS as the bearer of financial risk and the likely major player in the system.

When one curve is replaced by the other, it presents significant challenges for boards because they must not only accommodate, but also master the new curve or paradigm change. A *paradigm* is simply a mental model that provides leaders with boundaries for decision making and also gives rules for success by showing how to solve problems within the established boundaries. Paradigms act as screens, allowing boards to accept and respond to what is within the boundaries of the paradigm, what meets their expectations. Paradigms also force a board to reject anything that does not fit within the boundary, anything that is not within the board's realm of experience.

When a paradigm shifts, when the first curve yields to the second, everything changes. The old rules for success no longer work. In fact, following the old rules typically causes failure in the new reality of the second curve or shifted paradigm. For example, the incentives under managed care are diametrically opposed to those of fee for service. Attempting to survive in a managed care environment with a fee-for-service operating structure or leadership mind-set will lead to rapid and irreversible failure.

The transition to the new health care system will not be made easily because hospitals, and their boards, traditionally resist change. Consequently, they usually are swept along or rolled over by change and rarely influence, control, manage, or direct the change that will dictate their future.

There are many reasons why boards typically resist change. For example, a board may be comfortable with the old paradigm, the first curve, and in its complacency does not wish to change. Some boards, realizing that they must change, do not know how and become paralyzed into inaction; others deny that change is occurring; and still others fear change.

One fundamental reason that boards tend to resist change is a result of how they spend their time and structure their agenda (discussed in greater detail in chapter 4). In the first curve, when things are stable and prosperous, a typical health care organization board spends most of its time monitoring the past. Its agenda is largely consumed with discussion of what happened last month, last quarter, or last year. This type of governance "by looking into the rearview mirror" tends to perpetuate the past rather than prepare a board to address the future.

When confronted with the advent of a second curve or a new paradigm, an effective board realizes that spending a majority of its time monitoring the past is inappropriate and, in fact, dangerous. Effective boards must spend their time creating the future, not monitoring the past. Put another way:

> Board meetings are for creating the future, not for hearing reports about last month nor for ritualistically approving decisions that could as well have been finalized by management. Governance is not about budget lines, benefit plans or reacting to administrative initiatives. It is about empowering an organization toward visionary but attainable results within crafted boundaries.[4]

Effective boards control how they spend their time. When approaching or in the early stages of a new curve or paradigm, a board should spend the majority of its time deliberating and planning the future. Talking about the past (monitoring) should be reduced to no more than 25 percent of a board's time, and talking about and creating the future (planning, setting policy, and making decisions) should consume a majority, or about 75 percent, of a board's time. Boards must drive their organizations by spending most of their time looking forward through the windshield, not backward into the rearview mirror.

Effective health care organization boards must become change masters. To do this, they must be opened up to a series of structured inquiries, a raising of key questions that will cause them to explore new ideals and approaches; and they must develop and pursue new objectives for their organizations.

However, before boards can be change masters of their organizations, they must be change masters of themselves. Before a board can hope to successfully manipulate the levers to create and lead an IDS, it must be able to successfully manipulate the levers that control the process, function, and structure of governance.

What are the governance levers that boards must control? The four most important ones are:

1. How board members spend their time together
2. How a board controls and structures its agenda
3. How a board controls and structures the information it receives

4. How a board structures itself (such as its committee structure and its composition)

When a board controls these four critical governance levers, it will then be able to control the fifth crucial governance lever: how a board makes decisions.

Health care organization boards need to respond to the massive and rapid changes in health care by taking action that is inherently risky to their organizations. In fact, the market favors those organizations with a bias for action ("fortune favors the brave"). Boards caught in the old monitoring paradigm of governance will be frustrated in their attempts to do this. Boards that redesign the process and structure of governance to control the levers of governance will be best prepared to lead their organizations into the future.

Before boards embark on reevaluating their function and structure to achieve more meaningful governance, they can benefit from consideration of the context in which they govern. The next chapter discusses a context for effective governance in health care systems. It emphasizes a systems-thinking approach to leadership and key relationships that define the governance arena in IDSs.

References

1. The Governance Institute. *Governance Trends and Practices in Hospitals: 1994 Panel Survey of Hospitals.* La Jolla, CA: The Governance Institute, 1994.
2. The Governance Institute. *Governance Trends and Practices in Health Systems: 1995 Panel Survey of System Boards.* La Jolla, CA: The Governance Institute, 1995.
3. Morrison, I. The two-curve problem: high-risk challenges face those who plan a hospital's future. *The Baxter Foundation's Health Management Quarterly* 16(1):11, First Quarter 1994.
4. Carver, J. To focus on shaping the future, many hospital boards might require a radical overhaul. *The Baxter Foundation's Health Management Quarterly* 16(1):7, First Quarter 1994.

Chapter 3

A Context for Governance in Systems

Just as the changing health care environment stimulates and provides a context for development of integrated delivery systems (IDSs), systems themselves motivate and become the context for governance transformation. Boards that seek to transform themselves to govern systems more effectively cannot do so successfully in a vacuum. Determining the appropriate function of governance and the best structure to support that function fundamentally depends on a clear understanding of the context for governance in systems.

This chapter suggests that effective governance depends on a systems-thinking approach. In other words, boards must think and act in terms of what is best for the system, rather than for its components. The chapter also discusses key competencies that all boards must exercise in order to govern effectively and focuses in greater detail on the development, nurturing, and management of key relationships that are the essence of IDSs and therefore the context within which IDS boards govern.

Becoming a Systems Thinker

Individual organizations that successfully join together to form a new whole transform themselves in the process. They come to realize that what might be good for one part of the organization might not be good for the organization as a whole and that working together to reach a common goal is the way to achieve results.

For most organizations, the transformation from autonomy to interdependence is a necessary and difficult journey. Those organizations that find success often are stimulated, motivated, and guided by leaders whose vision is a whole greater than the sum of its parts—whose leadership and oversight is directed at the interconnected system of people, relationships, and organizations, rather than at any individual or part.

Leaders who transform organizations from parts into a greater whole are *systems thinkers*.

Systems thinking is a discipline for seeing wholes.[1] Characteristics of systems thinking include:

- Seeking harmony in interaction
- Balancing analysis (examination of parts) with synthesis (seeing the parts as a whole)
- Painting the whole picture, with all parts, big and small
- Emphasizing patterns of change over time rather than static snapshots of behavior or activity
- Pursuing root causes of behavior to avoid symptomatic solutions
- Focusing on integration and interconnectedness and on interrelationships, rather than linear cause-and-effect chains

Systems thinking identifies the interdependencies that drive behavior and enables leaders to select high-leverage interventions for lasting results. It is a framework for understanding the world around us that identifies and examines key interrelationships among variables and the patterns these relationships are part of over time. Once the patterns are clear and a common understanding of them is shared among leaders and within the organization, it is possible to alter their structure effectively to achieve new behaviors and goals. In fact, a belief in our ability to alter the structures in which we operate is an important and necessary first step in organizational transformation.

Systems thinkers understand that individuals and institutions can and must be the architects of their own reality in order to structure an environment that is most conducive to future survival and success. However, although many organizations are now creating integrated structures designed to seamlessly provide an array of services, they are finding that structure itself is just the tip of the iceberg. For systems to deliver on their promise of several interconnected, interdependent organizations working as one, the concept of being a system must move beyond a paper structure to a way of thinking and acting that makes the system the focal point, rather than any one subsidiary organization or individual.

Becoming a systems thinker can be a difficult transition because traditional loyalty to one institution must be set aside and replaced with loyalty to the system. This necessary shift in focus has important implications for everyone in the system but especially for system leaders, who must embrace the shift and ensure that it is understood and implemented throughout the organization. What follows is a discussion of several mental blinders to systems thinking and some ideas on how to overcome them.

- *My reality is the reality.* We all see the world from our own sometimes unique perspectives, yet we all know where the world would be if no one considered other possibilities. For example, without Christopher Columbus we might still believe that the world is flat. If Galileo had not dared to believe that the earth orbited the sun, we would still be in the Dark Ages.

In the modern world, we have direct evidence that one phenomenon can actually have completely different physical properties: Light is both a particle and a wave. Further, we know that Newtonian physics and quantum physics both work, yet disagree in principle. Therefore, reality often is a function of our own point of view. The danger lies in believing that our own reality is the only reality or the only correct way to perceive the world.

Systems thinkers entertain and learn to move comfortably among many realities. Board members or leaders who cannot see the bigger picture but, rather, remain focused on the organization they originally led or governed may well miss making decisions that are right for the future because they cannot conceptualize or embrace alternatives. Closing a flagship institution, partnering with your biggest competitor or "enemy," and focusing on maintaining health rather than treating illness all are ways of operating that are very different from the ways health care organizations have operated in the past. Systems thinkers know that doing the same things better is no longer good enough. Doing new things, and continuously doing them better, is the way to create a new and functional reality.

- *Separating self from external reality.* In the face of rapid change such as the health care field is now experiencing, it often is comfortable to divorce ourselves or our institution from what is happening "out there." This separation of self from the rest of the world creates a sense of disconnectedness that can have very serious implications for institutional survival. Such a view assumes that the organization has no influence on external circumstances or events and therefore must "play the hand it is dealt." Although it is easy to believe that change is happening *to* us, it is more productive to realize that change often is a direct consequence of our past actions. In other words, change happens *because* of us. For example, purchasers of health care are now spearheading the move to control health care costs. However, their actions are not occurring in a vacuum but, rather, are largely in response to a health care industry that historically has not monitored or attempted to control costs on its own.
- *Focusing on events rather than process.* This is a common pitfall that often is associated with outcomes management. Looking only at outcomes—and assigning blame when they are negative—prevents getting at the root cause of the problem, which frequently lies in the process or series of steps that produced the outcome. Systems

thinkers not only look at results, but also seek to understand why those results occurred. They understand that cause and effect often are separated by time and space. Therefore, when evaluating results, systems thinkers ask how outcomes were achieved, what needs to change in the process, and how long the change will take.

Systems thinkers also understand that near-term pain may mean longer-term gain and that old indicators of success may signal less-positive outcomes in a new reality. For example, as organizations switch from providing acute inpatient care to managed care or capitation, daily hospital census probably will decline. Living with decreasing inpatient revenue may well be part of the switch to managed care, and hospital leaders should be willing to set old notions aside and interpret this indicator as a part of the change as they look for evidence of growth on the outpatient side. Given outpatient growth, declining inpatient census may actually signal a positive change for a system moving toward lower-cost outpatient care.

- *Fragmentation thinking.* Systems thinkers know that the whole is greater than the sum of its parts and that it can produce an outcome that surpasses any results generated by individual units. Therefore, systems thinkers realize that no one part of the system is more important than any other. In a true system, neither the hospital, its chief executive officer (CEO), nor a particular group of physician specialists or founding board members are more important than the system itself; and the needs of individuals or specific entities should be eclipsed by the needs of the system. This overriding sense of the whole also makes systems thinkers continuously ask how activities conducted by one part of the system affect the rest of the system. They know that each entity must act to maximize the good of the system as a whole and that allocation of resources and other decisions that are made for one unit should be evaluated primarily against the effect they will have on the system and not made to maximize the results for that unit alone.
- *The enemy is out there.* Just as we sometimes think that we are controlled by external events, we also tend to define ourselves in terms of our worst threats or enemies. The United States today has been described as being in the throes of an identity crisis because our traditional enemy, the Soviet Union, has dissolved and we can no longer define ourselves as that nation's antithesis. Systems thinkers strive to create an identity for their organization that is independent of external threats. In a world where one's worst enemy may now be one's most advantageous partner, organizations must have a clear sense of who they are so that they can identify and achieve their own goals.

- *Big change requires big action.* Some organizations never get off the mark because they assume that only big, sweeping action will produce the major changes being called for in today's environment. Leaders of organizations that are well on their way to functioning effectively as systems point to just the opposite approach as the key to success. Taking a series of well-focused steps over time will produce significant change. Lasting, meaningful change cannot occur overnight, largely because of the nature of organizations, as discussed below.
- *The organization is like a machine.* Organizations are organic, living systems. Thus change is best assimilated, rather than imposed. Indeed, organizations, like the people who comprise them, do not easily accept changes thrust on them. Education, preparation, and periodic reinforcement and support are necessary to assist organizations to make transitions successfully.
- *The illusion of control.* Change makes us realize that we have no absolute control over our environment. Although control is comfortable, the realization that total control is impossible can actually free organizations to take risks and move ahead, rather than be paralyzed by the fear of making a wrong move. Systems thinkers understand that through change there is opportunity to influence the environment for the benefit of the organization.

How many of these barriers to systems thinking affect your board or organization? Board members and other organizational leaders who understand common impediments to systems thinking not only can work to overcome them, but also can be alert to their occurrence within the system and take steps to ensure that they do not get in the way of achieving system goals. Board members who overcome these obstacles and apply systems thinking to their leadership really can create the future, as the following case example illustrates.

An Example of Systems Thinking in Governance

South Suburban Hospital, located in Hazel Crest, Illinois, is a 250-bed, not-for-profit hospital with a community board. Although the hospital was doing well financially, with a strong bottom line and healthy reserves, through a strategic planning process the board realized that the Chicago-area health care market would soon change from one largely composed of individual institutions to one composed of a few large health care systems. Even though the hospital was positioned to continue to do well financially for several years, well after the terms of many current board members expired, the board and the hospital's CEO, Bob Rutkowski, developed an affiliation strategy and began to aggressively identify and seek partners. Discussions ensued, and in December 1994, the board voted to affiliate with Evangelical Health System (EHS). (To illustrate how quickly markets can change, even as South Suburban was in affiliation discussions with EHS, EHS merged with the Lutheran General System to form Advocate Health System.)

Following is an excerpt from a letter written by a member of the South Suburban board to one of the authors of this book, James E. (Jamie) Orlikoff, who also was a member of the South Suburban board during the affiliation process.[2] This letter illustrates the challenge of translating systems thinking into action.

> December 5, 1994
>
> Dear Jamie:
>
> I left the board meeting the other night with many strong feelings. I felt satisfied with the result of our vote to affiliate with EHS. Patients, employees, and physicians for years to come will benefit from our efforts.
>
> I felt a shared sense of commitment to the future of the hospital and its new partners. That commitment is strong because we worked diligently, selflessly, and, I believe, covered all the bases. That commitment will make it work.
>
> I also felt a sense of loss. We won't have the same control that we and our predecessors respected and exercised. It is satisfying to know, however, that we chose to take the control away from ourselves. . . .
>
> Sincerely,
>
> Sam Ogrizovich, CFP

As the letter illustrates, South Suburban's board was able to overcome several blinders to systems thinking. Among these were:

- *The illusion of control.* The board realized that it would need to give up its control to assure the future and achieve the mission of the organization.
- *The enemy is out there.* The board realized that other systems, instead of being just competitors, could also be potential partners.
- *My reality is the reality.* The board could have ignored the changing market and focused only on the hospital's current financial

health, projecting that scenario into the future and denying the impact that the market would eventually have on the hospital.

As systems thinkers, the South Suburban board members and CEO understood that the hospital was part of a bigger system (the Chicago-area health care market), and as a component of that system, it was interconnected with, and affected by, other system components. The board and CEO also understood that relationships among components of a system change over time. Because the CEO and board were aware of these interdependencies, they could identify and implement strategies for the hospital that would help ensure its continued viability for the future. In so doing, the board effectively altered the structure of the bigger system to achieve new goals, even when that action resulted in less control for the hospital's board. As systems thinkers, board members kept their focus on the bigger picture, rather than on only one of its parts.

Systems Thinking and Community Health: A Case Example

It is interesting that the words *whole* and *health* come from the same root word, the Old English *hal* as in "hale and hearty."[3] The implication is that perceiving the whole helps us to create or foster health. As health care leaders, we are challenged to perceive ever-greater wholes, to think beyond our health care organizations or systems and see them, in effect, as part of a larger system—a healthy community. The following case example can help us stretch our leadership context and apply systems thinking to improve community health.

An increasing leadership focus on healthy communities and community accountability reflects a changing dynamic in health care. Yet, it often is easier to talk about community health than it is for health care leaders to protect and improve it. A case in point is the Chicago heatwave deaths in 1995.

On July 12–16, the city of Chicago experienced a record heat wave with daily maximum temperatures ranging between 93 and 106 degrees Fahrenheit and minimum evening temperatures never falling below the low 90s. The more than 600 deaths attributed to the heat wave were double the number of deaths attributed to the Great Chicago Fire of 1871. More than 60 percent of the dead were over 65 years of age, with an average age of 72. According to the Centers for Disease Control and Prevention, heat-related deaths are "readily preventable," especially as the first deaths did not occur until the end of the second day of the heat wave. However, to implement effective preventive measures, the causes of the heat-related deaths must be known.

In this case, there was no single cause of the fatal epidemic. Rather, the Chicago heat-related deaths were a consequence of the unique systemic interaction of atmospheric, demographic, industrial, medical, urban design, and socioeconomic variables. In addition to the high heat, unusually high humidity created a heat index of as much as 119. The concrete environment of the city absorbed, radiated, and magnified the heat. The high ozone pollution levels added to the biological stress on Chicagoans' cardiovascular and pulmonary systems. Many elderly were without air-conditioning and refused to leave their homes to seek it due to fear of crime, even though they were encouraged to do so by the city and social service organizations. In fact, many of the dead were found in homes with closed and locked doors and windows, suggesting that their fear of crime prevented them from even ventilating their homes. The breakdown of the extended family structure left many elderly without people to check on them and provide support. Certain common medications, such as tranquilizers and diuretics, made the elderly more vulnerable by reducing their sensitivity to heat as well as their bodies' ability to regulate heat.

This community health problem is not just a one-time occurrence confined to Chicago. Many fatalities were reported in Kansas City and St. Louis during a 1980 heat wave and in Philadelphia when a heat wave hit that city in 1993. If global warming is indeed a reality, more heat waves and heat mortality epidemics can be expected in the future.

How can health care leaders concerned with assessing and improving the health of their communities address this issue? Because epidemic heat mortality is not due to a single cause, effective health care leaders will not seek a single solution. Rather, they will work to fashion a system of solutions to address the many complex and interrelated etiologic variables. Finally, they will work to understand exactly what a healthy community is.

According to a recent study by the Healthcare Forum, the critical determinants of a healthy community are:[4]

1. Low crime rate
2. Good place to raise children
3. Low level of child abuse
4. Not afraid to walk late at night
5. Good schools
6. Strong family life
7. High environmental quality
8. Good jobs and a healthy economy
9. High-quality health care
10. Affordable health care

Health care leaders must learn from the Chicago experience that community health is not a single event or issue, and that everything is related to everything else.

Developing a Leadership Action Plan

Imagine that a severe heat wave is predicted for your community this summer. Your organization has several months to prepare and is determined that one of the first steps ought to be development of a leadership action plan. Using the systems-thinking principles discussed above and the questions that follow, construct such an action plan:

1. Beyond the elderly, who will be clearly at risk during the predicted heat wave? What other populations in your community might be at risk as well?
2. What special needs will the different at-risk populations have? What resources and actions will best address these needs?
3. What organizations in the community might work together to provide needed services and resources?
4. With which of these organizations does your health care organization already have relationships?
5. How might your organization effectively collaborate with these and other potential partners to plan and execute necessary activities?
6. How does your organization and its partners define your *community*?
7. What determinants of a healthy community from the Healthcare Forum study discussed above does your community possess? What impact, if any, might these determinants have on development of your action plan?
8. What role and level of accountability will your organization's leaders have for maximizing community health during the predicted heat wave?
9. How will the overall success of the plan and its execution be evaluated?

Although systems thinking can be applied effectively to deal with a health-related crisis such as a heat wave, its potential to provide a framework for assessing and improving overall community health is clear. Understanding the interdependencies among people and organizations, and the need to focus on the whole rather than a snapshot of its parts, along with the willingness to change the way we think about our world and how we interact with it, and the willingness to focus on underlying causes rather than symptoms can provide a strong foundation for the collaborative, creative efforts necessary to deal with a complex, multivariate issue such as community health. Such qualities also provide perhaps the only constructive framework within which to take meaningful steps to improve community health.

Key Skills and Competencies

In addition to adopting a systems-thinking approach to governance, effective boards not only have a clear sense of their roles and responsibilities—the core of governance—but also understand the skills and competencies they must exercise as they govern. Whether engaged in mission stewardship, operational oversight, strategic goal setting, policy development, or any other aspect of governance, effective boards exhibit and continue to develop the following characteristics and competencies:

- *Emphasis on mission and values:* The board understands and accommodates the culture and values of the organization it governs, and reflects these in the mission.
- *Education and performance improvement:* The board ensures that trustees are well informed about the institution, the field, and the board's roles, responsibilities, and performance.
- *Loyalty to the board as a group:* The board supports development of the trustees as a group, focuses on the collective welfare of the board, and develops a sense of group cohesiveness.
- *Emphasis on the big picture:* The board relies on multiple perspectives to analyze complex problems and generate appropriate responses. It understands its fundamental oversight and policy-setting role and does not engage in management or operational decision making.
- *Fostering relationships with key constituencies:* The board accepts as a primary responsibility the need to develop and maintain healthy relationships among key constituencies.
- *Strategic thinking and direction setting:* The board helps envision and shape institutional direction and helps ensure a strategic approach to the organization's future.

Although specific aspects of many of these competencies are discussed in chapter 4, relationships among key constituencies are discussed here because they provide a practical context for system governance. If, as suggested in chapter 1, an integrated delivery system (IDS) is fundamentally a complex and interdependent set of relationships, boards must be able to identify, develop, manage, and nurture these relationships in order to govern successfully.

Key Governance Relationships

The following relationships define a context for governance in systems:

- Board–mission relationship
- Board–CEO relationship
- Board–physician entity relationships
- Relationships among trustees and boards
- Board–community relationships

Each of these is addressed in the following subsections.

Board–Mission Relationship

Whether a hospital, a multihospital system, or an IDS, the primary purpose of governance is the same: to steer the organization toward accomplishment of its mission. The mission statement is the cornerstone of all of the organization's activities and relationships. It is also the cornerstone of the operation of the board.

A constant of effective governance is the ultimate accountability of the board to the mission of the organization or system it governs. This provides a context for effective governance even as governance changes shape and function.

The mission is both the governance and system rudder. The most fundamental governance responsibility and function is mission stewardship: to develop a meaningful mission statement, to routinely evaluate the mission to verify that it is still valid, to modify it when appropriate, and to ensure that the plans and practices of the system and its boards are consistent with the mission.

A focus on mission and governance function results in more emphasis placed on how and why governance decisions are made and less emphasis on how governance is structured. Unfortunately, the mission statements of most systems are so general as to be useless in that they provide no system definition and outline no direction for it. In such situations, governance has abdicated its responsibility to develop a meaningful mission. Consequently, the board does not have a mission to follow as it governs the system and will find itself without a guiding light during times of crisis and at critical decision points, such as determining the philosophy and structure of governance. Thus, governance function becomes hazy, and in an attempt to seek clarity and meaning, governance structure often becomes the focus.

Without a mission focus, governance tends to naturally regress to an institutional or representational focus. In other words, instead of focusing on the mission, the board(s) focuses on the best financial interests of the system, or of its component parts, which are not always congruent with the mission. This is true regardless of how system board members are chosen. The converse also is true: A board selected from representative components of the system will not necessarily function as a representative board if its members have a mission focus.

Consider this hypothetical situation. A man comes before your board with a briefcase filled with magic pills, offering to sell them for 15 cents each. He claims that those people who take the pill will never again experience illness or injury, and existing disease would be cured. The board is asked whether it wishes to buy the pills and give one to each person in the community.

If your board distributes the pills to the community, the hospital or system could well go out of business. On the other hand, if the board buys the pills and destroys them, or charges an exorbitant sum for them, the institution would profit and continue to exist, but would do so at the expense of the community. What should the board do? What should guide the board in making its decision? The answer to both questions should be found in the mission of the organization.

Effective governance requires an effective mission. Why? In tough and turbulent times, a board without a clear sense of organizational purpose is likely to focus on short-term issues, overreact to events, and contribute to organizational drift and disarray. Further, the board is more likely to focus on the internal organization (its financial viability and growth) than on the external community and constituents.

The mission is the primary force that holds an organization together. Thus, validity of the mission and the degree to which the organization is successful in achieving it must be the board's central concern. Effective governance requires an effective mission. But what is an effective mission?

Following is a compelling definition of the mission and its importance:

> The mission focuses the organization on action. It defines the specific strategies needed to attain the crucial goals. It creates a disciplined organization. It alone can prevent the most common degenerative disease of organizations . . . splintering their always limited resources.[5]

A mission defines what the organization is and what it is not. A key characteristic of a good mission is that it helps board members make difficult decisions by giving them a guiding set of principles with which to operate and make decisions.

A mission should be current, relevant, and specific enough to position the system or hospital uniquely within its service area. To help ensure that the mission clearly and precisely states the hospital's reason for being, it should identify the purpose, philosophy, and perhaps the values of the organization and should include a focus on the health needs of the community. A mission can have the following components:

- Type of organization: Teaching, government, religious
- Scope of services: Long-term, acute, continuum of care (exclusions, if any)
- Service area definition/intended customers: City, county, region, particular demographic group (women, children, cancer or tuberculosis patients)
- Type or dimensions of care: Spiritual, psychological
- Strengths, limitations: Cost, access, quality, special affiliations
- Community focus

What are the right questions for boards to ask in developing and maintaining a viable mission? Consider the following:

- What is our belief system?
- Who are our customers?
- What is our job?

These questions are fundamental to establishing an organization's mission and can be useful as a basic checklist for helping to ensure mission-based governance. For example, a health care system may be faced with a decision to establish a health plan. The board might pose the following questions: How would the health plan fit with our organization's basic beliefs and values? Does owning a health plan make the most sense given the population we serve? Is bearing the risk of financing as well as delivering care consistent with what we do or ought to do as an organization? What are the pros and cons of other alternatives?

Professor Regina E. Herzlinger of the Harvard Business School also recommends four questions central to governance that have emerged from her 25 years of studying nonprofit organizations:[6]

1. Are the organization's goals consistent with its financial resources?
2. Is the organization practicing intergenerational equity, that is, are future users of the organization's programs and services treated fairly or kept in mind in decisions the organization makes today?
3. Are sources and uses of funds appropriately matched?
4. Is the organization sustainable?

Many of these questions support the adage "No margin, no mission." They deal with whether the organization has the financial resources necessary to support its mission and whether these resources are allocated appropriately. The question of "intergenerational equity" is particularly relevant in today's environment of constrained resources and begs the converse of the above adage: No mission, no margin. More than ever, careful, thoughtful deployment of limited resources is essential to ensuring that the right health care is available at the right place and time to meet the health care needs of the population served today and into the future. Without a clear understanding of its identity and purpose, an organization risks using resources in ways that do not further its mission and goals, resulting in potential loss of focus, market position, and competitive advantage.

Boards are increasingly confronted with questions about what is best for the long term. Thinking in terms of what best meets the overall health care needs of the community today and tomorrow can help a board make tough decisions, such as those involving relocation or reduction of services. A long-term perspective also helps leaders view some decisions, such as whether to merge or affiliate or whether to focus on health maintenance rather than treatment of illness, as opportunities rather than threats.

With all the dizzying changes in health care and hospitals, it is an appropriate time for most boards to ask: Is our mission still relevant? Many well-known organizations have examined and revised their missions and in doing so have changed their identities and continued to exist with a new focus. Many different situations can precipitate a revision of an organization's mission. These include fulfillment of the original mission; a change in market conditions, such as the emergence of unmet needs, or unnecessary and wasteful duplication of services; new industry trends; systemic restructuring of financial and/or delivery systems; new legislative requirements or initiatives; and many others.

Many of these situations are present or likely to emerge in the near future in the health care environment. Thus, many health care organizations may need a revised mission in order to remain relevant and viable.

An effective board envisions the purpose of its organization and from this shapes a strategic direction to help ensure that the organization achieves it. The board envisions the purpose of the organization through the mission and through the mission creates the future for the organization.

Board–CEO Relationship

The CEO is the board's primary link to the organization; thus, the board's relationship with the CEO is one of its most important responsibilities. (See the effective governance pyramid in figure 4-1, p. 41.) Selecting, evaluating, and retaining the right CEO for an integrated health care system can be among the board's biggest challenges and requires a clear sense of the skills, expertise, and leadership attributes that will be required for success in the new organization. Executive recruiters suggest several important traits of successful leaders in integrated systems:[7]

- The ability to articulate a concise strategy and how to implement it
- The willingness to share power with other constituencies, especially physicians
- The ability to articulate objectives and demand results
- The ability to know when things are not working and to change course
- The capability to negotiate, not dictate
- Physical and mental health

Whether the board chooses for the system CEO the CEO of an existing organization that will be folded into the new system or launches a search for a new top executive, these characteristics for success can help provide guidance, not only for selecting but also for evaluating and retaining appropriate talent.

The challenges of running a multiorganizational system often are more complex and long-term than those facing a single organization, and such challenges likely will require new types and levels of performance from the organization's top executives. Therefore, system boards must be keenly attuned to the need to set clear expectations and to provide ongoing feedback and evaluation and appropriate rewards and recognition for a health care system's chief executive. More and more, these responsibilities are being assigned to a compensation committee of the board. This committee ensures that the organization's compensation philosophy ties into the system's overall strategic objectives and that the CEO evaluation process is comprehensive, up-to-date, and functioning properly for all participants. A sample compensation committee charter appears in figure 3-1 and outlines the composition and responsibilities for such a committee. Assigning CEO selection, evaluation, development, and rewards to a specific board committee can help provide the appropriate level of focus and attention to this board responsibility to ensure that the system's top executive is properly prepared, motivated, and supported to achieve the system's strategic goals.

Board–Physician Entity Relationships

Integrated systems typically have a variety of relationships with physicians that often transcend the traditional relationship with the medical staff. A thorough discussion of physician–hospital organizations, medical services organizations, foundations, and the myriad other relationships that are evolving between health care organizations and physicians

Figure 3-1. Sample Compensation Committee Charter

The Compensation Committee of the Board of Directors shall consist of not less than three nor more than six outside members of the Board of Directors, one of whom shall be the chairperson. The committee and its chairperson shall be elected annually by the Board of Directors.

The Board of Directors delegates to the Compensation Committee strategic and administrative responsibility for a broad range of issues. The committee's basic responsibility is to assure that the Chief Executive Officer, other officers, and key management of the organization are compensated effectively in a manner consistent with the stated compensation strategy of the organization, internal equity considerations, competitive practice, and the requirements of appropriate regulatory bodies. The committee shall also communicate to stakeholders the organization's compensation policies and the reasoning behind such policies.

More specifically, the committee shall be responsible for the following:

1. Review annually and approve the organization's stated compensation strategy to ensure that management is rewarded appropriately for its contributions to organization growth and profitability and that the executive compensation strategy supports organization objectives and stakeholder interests.

2. Review annually and determine the individual elements of total compensation for the Chief Executive Officer and communicate in the annual Board Compensation Committee Report the factors and criteria on which the Chief Executive Officer's compensation for the last year was based, including the relationship of the organization's performance to the Chief Executive Officer's compensation.

3. Review and approve the individual elements of total compensation for the executive officers and key management other than the Chief Executive Officer and communicate in the annual Board Compensation Committee Report the specific relationships of organization performance to executive compensation.

4. Assure that the annual incentive compensation plan is administered in a manner consistent with the organization's compensation strategy and the terms of the plan as to the following:
   - Participation
   - Target annual incentive awards
   - Organization financial goals
   - Actual awards paid
   - Total funds reserved for payment under the plan

Figure 3-1. (Continued)

> 5. Approve all new longer-term incentive plans for management and administer the organization's long-term incentive programs in a manner consistent with the terms of the plans as to the following:
>   - Participation
>   - Vesting requirements
>   - Awards
>   - Total compensation reserved for awards
>
> 6. Approve an annual aggregate amount that may be used by the Chief Executive Officer for special incentive awards.
>
> 7. Approve revisions to the organization's salary range structure, salary increase guidelines, and executive promotions.
>
> 8. Review with the Chief Executive Officer compensation matters relating to management succession.
>
> 9. Review the organization's employee benefit programs and approve changes subject, where appropriate, to Board of Director approval.
>
> 10. Assure that the CEO evaluation process is based on mutually established expectations and goals, provides for frequent and ongoing review, and addresses both executive performance and development.

Source: Adapted from KPMG Peat Marwick. Assessment of executive compensation—guidelines for the compensation committee. *Compensation Briefs* (93-1):5–6, Feb. 1993.

are beyond the scope of this book. Yet, regardless of the number or types of relationships between a health care system and its physicians, effective system boards see physicians as leadership partners involved in all aspects of system oversight and operation, including governance, clinical care and decision making, system management, strategic planning, managed care, quality improvement, community relations, and a variety of other activities.

Boards that have successful leadership partnerships with physicians involve physician leaders early on in strategic planning and decision making and ensure that physician and organizational goals and incentives are clarified and aligned. They ensure that the organization communicates regularly with physicians and commits the resources necessary to provide educational opportunities that help support and develop physicians as leaders and executives. Boards also realize that retaining power means giving power, including shared control and ownership.

Relationships among Trustees and Boards

The multiple-board structure of many IDSs is making coordination of governance activities more complex. As parent and subsidiary boards emerge with different roles and responsibilities, systems are challenged to ensure that each board has the appropriate membership, structure, and support to effectively discharge its duties and to understand how it fits into overall system governance. In addition, a variety of communication, education, and other initiatives are being used in systems between and among boards to help build an effectively functioning governance infrastructure.

Organizations that fail to provide necessary coordination and support for governance often find their boards to be top heavy or dysfunctional. Ways of functionally dealing with relationships among system trustees and boards, along with issues relating to the structure of these relationships, are discussed in chapter 4. Specific approaches to the various structural models of governance are discussed in chapter 5.

Board–Community Relationships

As markets and other forces drive systemic reform, communities are becoming the focal point for change in health care. With the growth of managed care and capitation, financial incentives have shifted away from sickness care to reward providers for maintaining the health of enrolled populations, or covered lives. Effective health care leaders realize that the overall community will affect the health of their organization's enrollees and are therefore shifting their focus toward maintaining and improving overall community health.

System boards that seek to have a meaningful impact on community health begin with a clear understanding of the specific "community" their health care organization serves and how this community is evolving and changing over time. As systems, health care organizations also should see themselves as part of the larger system of the community and understand the need to cultivate partnerships with other community organizations that can bring together diverse resources to help assess and improve community health status.

Health care system board members and other leaders can help to identify and develop these partnerships and clarify the shared vision, values, and plans necessary to support them in achieving their goals. System boards also can appoint a board committee to oversee the health care organization's role in such community initiatives, as well as the organization's own programs for community health.

Lastly, the goal of improved community health can only be achieved through clearly established accountability. Health care system boards should review the system's mission statement to ensure that it expresses the organization's commitment to community health. Accountability for community health improvement goals should become part of performance evaluation for both the system chief executive and the board through an ongoing board self-evaluation process.

Conclusion

Once board members achieve a common understanding of the context in which they are governing, they will be better equipped to function effectively. The next chapter outlines and discusses a framework for effective governance function that can be applied to any board or governance process within a health care system. Just as context supports function, so too does function dictate the most effective way to structure governance to achieve system goals.

References

1. Senge, P. M. *The Fifth Discipline: The Art and Practice of the Learning Organization.* New York City: Doubleday/Currency, 1990, p. 68.
2. Sam Ogrizovich, CFP, personal correspondence with James E. Orlikoff, Dec. 5, 1994.
3. Senge.
4. Healthcare Forum, National Civic League, and DYG, Inc. *What Creates Health? Individuals and Communities Respond.* San Francisco: Healthcare Forum, 1994.
5. Drucker, P. What business can learn from non-profits. *Harvard Business Review* 67(4):91, July–Aug. 1989.
6. Herzlinger, R. E. Effective oversight: a guide for nonprofit directors. *Harvard Business Review* 72(4):53, July–Aug. 1994.
7. Lloyd, J. S., and Hadelman, J. M. Retaining good leaders before and after mergers. *Trustee* 48(1):18, Jan. 1995.

Chapter 4

A Framework for Effective Governance

As discussed earlier, the more integrated a system is, the more likely it is to thrive. One of the key roles of governance, then, must be to lead systems toward full integration. However, this is not enough. To truly achieve the promised benefits of full-system integration, the system's governing body also must be willing and able to transform itself in the process of leading its system toward change and integration.

The Relationship between Governance Structure and Function

Although governance should be the engine that pulls the train of system integration, it often is, instead, the caboose dragging along behind. Even worse, the caboose often has the brakes on and hinders system integration and evolution. This is because many systems never adequately address the question of what the functions of governance are—in other words, what governance should do and how its functions should change as it evolves away from an institutional, acute care focus toward a continuum of services focus.

Several chapters in this book examine governance structure and outline techniques for streamlining it. Yet, it is important to bear in mind that governance structure, although essential, is nevertheless secondary to governance function. That is why this chapter, which is devoted to effective governance function, is presented before the chapters that address governance structure and restructuring techniques: Form follows function.

There is little agreement on the ideal governance structure for an integrated delivery system (IDS) or health care organization for a very good reason: System governance tends to, and should, reflect the historical and philosophical roots of the founding, sponsoring, or owning organizations. In other words, the characteristics that affect the function of governance also affect its structure.

The number of boards in a system, for example, often is regarded as a significant structural characteristic that critically affects governance function. However, it is important to remember that governance structure (issues such as numbers and sizes, decentralized or centralized boards, and governing body composition) does not in itself determine governance function. Structure can only facilitate or inhibit effective governance function. Thus, the proper structure for the governance of each system should be determined primarily by the unique and individually defined needs, culture, and mission of each system, which define its function.

Although governance structure and function will be tailored to individual health care organizations, effective governance relies on several common elements. Consider the following framework for effective governance, which applies to any board or governance process within a system, regardless of structure.

The Effective Governance Pyramid

As figure 4-1 shows, the process of effective governance can be depicted graphically as a pyramid. The base of the pyramid provides the foundation for each of the successive functions and activities. The farther up the pyramid a board progresses, the more effective the board it will be.

The Mission

The base of the effective governance pyramid is the mission of the system or organization. The mission (discussed in relation to governance in greater detail in chapter 3) is both the governance and system rudder. It defines the belief system of the board, forms the foundation for decision making, and provides direction for the system. The mission defines what the organization or system is and what it is not.

From a governance perspective, a key characteristic of a good mission is that it helps the board make difficult decisions. As stated in the mission, the values, philosophies, and beliefs that define the organization serve as touchstones that can help guide boards in making decisions that best support and fulfill the mission and therefore help the organization realize and express its identity and purpose. These touchstones then can be applied by the board in each situation it confronts. The result is a consistency and predictability in board decisions, which serves to integrate and align the disparate stakeholders associated with the system.

The most fundamental governance function is to develop a meaningful mission; and to routinely evaluate the mission to verify that it is still valid, to modify it when appropriate, and to ensure that the plans and practices of the system and its boards are consistent with the mission.

The Strategic Plan

Once a meaningful and clear mission has been developed, it should form the basis for development of the strategic plan. The mission establishes the parameters of strategy for the organization or system by creating boundaries and direction for the actions and operation of the system. The mission suggests the strategy, and the strategy reflects the mission. In other words, if an outsider were to review a system or health care organization's strategic plan, he or she should be able to infer its mission. Conversely, if an outsider were presented with the system's mission along with an environmental assessment, he or she should be able to roughly project the system's strategy.

Figure 4-1. Effective Governance Pyramid

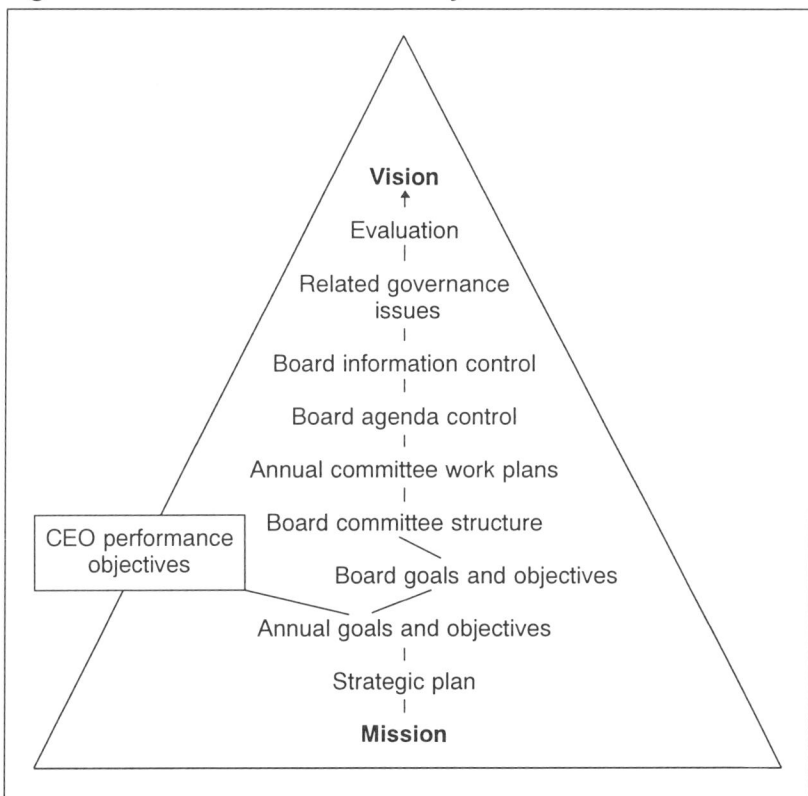

©Copyright 1996, Orlikoff & Associates, Chicago.

Thus, effective governance is framed by a dynamic tension between the mission and the strategic plan. Should a board find that it wishes to pursue a strategy that is inconsistent with the mission, it has two choices: It can either abandon the strategy and develop a new one consistent with the mission, or it can evaluate and revise the mission to accommodate the desired strategy.

An ineffective board will pursue strategy that is inconsistent with the mission and yet not revise the mission, preferring instead to maintain the illusion of the old mission while existing in the reality of a new, implicit mission. This creates a fundamental inconsistency between the formal belief system of the board (the explicit mission) and the actions of the organization as sanctioned by the board (the strategic plan). This results in an alienation of key stakeholders through a pattern of inconsistent governance decisions based on circumstance rather than principle. Unfortunately, this type of situational decision making is common among health care organization boards and condemns a board to a profound level of governance ineffectiveness.

The organization and oversight of strategic planning is therefore one of the most critical, but least effectively performed functions of system and health care organization boards. After mission inconsistency, another key reason that strategic planning tends to be ineffective is that it frequently focuses on perpetuating the past, rather than facilitating strategic thinking and action about the future.

Strategic planning is the process of determining what an organization should do, as well as when and how it should do it. Thus, strategic planning is really strategic thinking, strategic decision making, and strategic action. Effective strategic planning involves a series of complex steps. However, strategic planning is basically an organized process of determining how the system or organization will exist consistent with its mission and also meet the demands of changing present and future markets.

A common problem with many strategic planning processes arises from organizational denial—the inability or refusal of the board and other leaders to recognize and address the most critical issues confronting the system. (This has been referred to as "governance mural dyslexia," the inability of a board to read the handwriting on the wall!) As a result, many strategic plans identify and address dozens of minor issues but fail to address the one or two absolutely crucial issues. In other words, many plans nibble at the toes of the giant rather than strike at his heart.

As a board strives to ensure that the strategic direction is consistent with the mission and also is appropriate relative to the environment, it is important to remember that strategic plans are not static. Strategic planning involves evaluating and modifying existing plans and constantly developing new ones.

The purpose of strategic planning is not only to position the organization for the future but also, in a very real sense, to *create* the future for the organization. In order for the board to oversee such a process effectively, it is critical that the board be able to break the bounds of the past to effectively envision the future.

Annual Organizational Goals and Objectives

From the strategic plan will flow specific annual goals and objectives for the system. These goals and objectives are expressions of specific benchmarks of accomplishment that indicate effective implementation of the strategy. The goals and objectives are tactical in nature; they relate to how the strategy will be accomplished and incrementally measured. (Strategy relates to what will be done; tactics relate to how it will be done.)

As time horizons shorten for many strategic plans due to the volatile health care environment, many plans actually contain the system's annual goals and objectives. Whether the goals and objectives are contained in a separate document or within the strategic plan is not important. What is important is that the broad strategies are translated into specific, measurable goals and objectives. This is critical because these goals and objectives will form the basis for the focus of the board and the performance objectives for the chief executive officer (CEO).

Once the goals and objectives are developed, along with stated measures of goal/objective achievement, they must be operationalized. This is done through two related processes: development of the CEO performance objectives and development of the annual board goals and objectives. These are discussed in the next two sections.

CEO Performance Objectives

A classic question is: What is the difference between management and governance? Rather than ponder academic answers, this key question is best answered practically. Rather than arguing about the theoretical functions of the board and CEO, it is far more useful to distinctly organize their relative work.

The practical answer to the question of the difference between management and governance is determined for each CEO and board through development of distinct performance objectives for both. Specific and measurable annual CEO performance objectives should be based on the organization's annual goals and objectives, as well as on defined progress toward accomplishment of longer-term strategies and goals. This is the only meaningful way to focus CEO attention and activities on the system or organization's mission and strategic plan.

Unfortunately, in many health care organizations and systems, a dissonance frequently exists between organizational strategy and goals and CEO performance objectives. This is usually because the strategy is updated and changed whereas the CEO performance objectives are not. Unless this difference is reconciled with new CEO performance objectives, the CEO is placed in a veritable quandary. Should the CEO pursue achievement of the organization's strategy and risk being poorly evaluated due to failure to meet the old CEO performance objectives, or should he or she forget the performance objectives and prosecute the strategy in the hope that the board will disregard the old performance objectives when the CEO's performance is evaluated?

This is a very unhealthy situation for the CEO's career as well as for the system or organization's future. Only through a determined congruence between strategy, organizational goals and objectives, and CEO performance objectives can the board ensure that the CEO's time and attention is properly focused. Further, the progressive development of the CEO performance objectives also helps to protect the CEO against the considerable risk associated with doing his or her job properly.

Today's health care market conditions require CEOs who are willing to take bold and risky action. Yet, if the CEO is unsure of board support or does not know what the board expects of him or her, the CEO is more likely to play it safe, favoring short-term stability over long-term organizational survival.

Establishment of specific and measurable annual CEO performance objectives helps CEOs clearly understand the inexorable link between their performance and that of the system and organization. Further, it underscores the board's expectations of the CEO so that there is no confusion and no effort is wasted attempting to satisfy conflicting expectations or to divine nonexistent ones.

In addition, annual CEO performance objectives enable the board to:

- Link CEO compensation to CEO performance
- Provide an objective basis for recognizing and rewarding excellent performance
- Stay focused on stated roles, responsibilities, and functions of the CEO, and avoid implicit expectations
- Encourage CEO skill growth and development by creating a formal system to develop the CEO professionally and to help the CEO develop new and necessary skill sets and areas of expertise

This last point is an important one for board members to understand. The skill sets necessary to lead an IDS effectively are very different from those necessary to manage a hospital effectively. Thus, many hospital CEOs will need to develop new skills if they are to grow into effective

IDS CEOs. It is up to the board to ensure that its CEO is developing these new skills and that the annual CEO performance objectives are the vehicle to accomplish this development.

Annual CEO performance objectives can dramatically increase CEO willingness to take the risks necessary to create the viable health care system of the future. They help provide more structured, and therefore more stable, relationships between the CEO and the board by establishing clear distinctions between their respective roles. Because establishment of CEO performance objectives is so critical to achievement of organizational strategy and goals, many boards assign CEO selection, evaluation, and development to a separate committee of the board, typically the compensation committee. (See chapter 3.)

Annual Board Goals and Objectives

The preceding four progressive steps of the effective governance pyramid (mission, strategic plan, annual goals and objectives, and CEO performance objectives) are fairly straightforward from an organizational management perspective. They also form the springboard to effective governance function and structure.

As the annual organizational goals and objectives form the basis for CEO performance objectives, so too should they form the basis for annual board goals and objectives. Development of objectives for both the CEO and the board facilitates coordination and teamwork among the leadership of the organization or system. Although most boards understand the need for (if not actually develop) CEO performance objectives, few understand the need for or develop annual board goals and objectives.

When boards are asked during retreats whether they performed well during the past year, their response is almost always a resounding yes. When asked whether they had annual goals or objectives against which to measure their performance, boards almost always answer no. In effect, these boards are saying, "We don't know what our job is, but we did it very well!" When confronted with this restatement of their logic, most boards suddenly realize, like a ground glass lens brought sharply into focus, the value of annual board goals and objectives.

Just as CEO performance objectives focus the work, time, and attention of the CEO, so do annual board goals and objectives focus the work and structure of the board. In their absence, the temptation is strong for a board to think and act as if its work, meetings, and decisions are routine—the same from year to year. This is, in fact, why many boards regress into a stultifying sameness of function; even when there is environmental upheaval, the board does not perceive the need to modify its focus or function. Entrenched by the fear that usually accompanies change, this complacency, almost as if a board has been frozen in amber, is the antithesis of good governance.

In considering this, one of the key characteristics of effective governance emerges—that of a dynamic, evolving function and form. Effective governance ". . . must be elastic, able to stretch and adapt as circumstances warrant. Yet at the same time, it must be sufficiently resilient, disciplined, and self-aware" to change shape and function when conditions change.[1] The only disciplined way for a board to "stretch and adapt as circumstances warrant" is to do so within the context of structured goals and objectives that are explicitly developed on a regular basis to reflect changes in organizational focus and the environment.

It should be noted that annual CEO performance objectives and annual board objectives should be developed at the same time. Further, the board and the CEO should have input into both sets of objectives. This creates a formal "expectations exchange," where, through mutual discussion and negotiation, the board clarifies its expectations of the CEO and the CEO clarifies his or her expectations of the board. Once this is accomplished, the practical distinction between governance and management has been established.

Board Committee Structure

Only when specific board function has been determined is a board meaningfully prepared to address the issue of its structure. Once the board has developed its annual goals and objectives, it is then ready to determine its committee structure for the coming year. This is a new concept for most boards that exist with a "standing" committee structure, one that does not change from year to year. These boards often find themselves attempting to address 21st-century issues with a 1980s committee structure.

Such boards are likely to take one of three ineffective paths:

1. *Attempt to shoehorn new and challenging issues into a standing committee with a charge of overseeing past issues of diminishing importance.* For example, assign the issue of physician integration to the board medical staff relations committee. This approach almost always guarantees that new issues will not be addressed adequately and that the committees will continue to focus most of their attention on perpetuating the past rather than creating the future.
2. *Allow the outmoded standing committees to exist and concentrate on increasingly unimportant issues, while the board addresses new issues through formation of ad hoc committees.* Although this approach may allow the issues to be addressed, it also creates a top-heavy board

committee structure that requires board members to serve on, and management to staff, many committees. It also has the potential of creating a "two-class" board structure, with "important" (ad hoc) committees and "unimportant" (standing) committees.
3. *Create new committees to address new issues without eliminating any of the old standing committees.* This approach has the same disadvantages of the preceding path: It creates a top-heavy, two-class board committee structure that places excessive demands on both board member and management time. Further, over time, this approach results in an inordinate number of board committees because some boards find it easier to create new committees than to eliminate old ones.

All three of these common approaches to board committee structure and function are limited and limiting. A more effective approach is for each board to tailor its committee structure and function to the established priorities of the board—its goals and objectives. This can be accomplished through use of a "zero-based" board committee structure.

A *zero-based board committee structure* is one in which the board begins each year with a blank sheet of paper—in other words, no committees. Because the board has no committees, it must design them from scratch. The basis for committee design are the annual board goals and objectives.

For example, if, consistent with the strategy, a board goal and objective is to prepare to merge or affiliate with another organization to help facilitate formation of an IDS, the board might then create an affiliation committee. If a board goal and objective is to assess and improve the health of the community, a community health committee could be created. If a board goal and objective is to heavily invest in and use new information systems, an information technology committee could be created.

Frequently, a zero-based committee approach will result in several committees carrying over from year to year, such as finance, planning, quality, and an executive committee. (In addition, a governance or board development committee also may be warranted, as discussed at the end of this chapter.) However, the benefit of the exercise is that no committee's existence is taken for granted. Each existing committee is evaluated and continued or discontinued based on its relevance to accomplishing the stated annual board goals and objectives. The functions of several committees of the past year may be combined into one committee for the new year.

By using a zero-based board committee approach, a board is able to specifically tailor its committee structure to the major issues it will address—in other words, the priorities at hand. Further, by exercising the governance discipline of doing this each year, a board helps ensure that it is asking itself the tough questions and structuring itself so that it will function with maximum efficiency in, and be relevant to, a rapidly changing environment. This technique allows a board to avoid being trapped in a stultifying structure that paradoxically focuses its attention on past, increasingly irrelevant issues while the environment furiously changes.

Many boards have their specific committee structure mandated in the bylaws, and any change in committee structure requires a change in the bylaws. These boards are tempted to believe that they must rely on ad hoc committees if they wish to develop new board committees, as eliminating old or creating new committees requires amendments to the bylaws. Rather than amending the bylaws each year to accommodate the zero-based committee process, it is better to amend the bylaws once, and in the bylaws outline the zero-based committee process that will be followed each year by the board.

Annual Board Committee Work Plans

If a board does not control its committees, the committees will control it. As outlined in the preceding section, boards must exercise control over their committee structure, or what committees they have. Equally important, boards must control the focus and activities of the committees, or what the committees do.

Most boards do not control their committees but, rather, are controlled by them. This is because most boards, in addition to not controlling their committee structure, do not provide their committees with direction, focus, or specific tasks; they do not control what the committees do. In this case, the board is investing each board committee chair with responsibility for developing an implicit work plan and focus for the committee.

When a board relies on a committee chair to establish the committee direction, three things are likely to result: First, he or she will simply follow the lead of the previous committee chair. This approach perpetuates the past and locks the board into a limited pattern of functioning. Second, the committee chair will do what he or she wants to do with the committee. This may be appropriate if he or she has a good sense of where the board is going and how the committee fits into the big picture, but it usually results in each board committee going in a different direction, fragmenting the board's work and energy. Third, he or she relies on management to supply direction for the committee.

Each of these approaches is inappropriate and inhibits the board from functioning effectively. The board must direct all of its committees in order to align their direction and function so that the board can achieve its annual goals and objectives, and through that, accomplish the system or organization's goals and objectives, strategy, and mission. This type of organizational alignment is absolutely critical if the board is to make efficient use of its time and function at peak effectiveness.

To accomplish this, the board (once it has determined the annual committee structure through the zero-based process) must provide each committee with an annual committee work plan. This document outlines the committee's tasks, responsibilities, and functions; and establishes specific priorities and measurable objectives the committee is to address and accomplish.

For example, a board with an annual objective of identifying potential affiliation partners would be interested in developing and applying criteria to identify the best potential candidates. This board might then make development of such criteria a high priority for several of its committees. For example, the finance committee might be assigned the task of developing six financial criteria, the quality committee the task of developing six quality-related criteria, and so on. Additionally, assuming that as part of its affiliation objective the board also wants to "dress up" the organization to make it an attractive affiliation or merger partner, the board also might assign each committee the task of identifying strengths and weaknesses in organizational areas and recommending for board approval specific strategies to improve the weaknesses.

In this way, a board exercises specific control over each of its committees, ensures that the committee work is facilitating the efficient accomplishment of board goals and objectives, and minimizes the wasted time and effort on the part of board members and management that so often is associated with board committee function.

Board Agenda Control

The single most precious commodity a board possesses is the time its members spend together. In fact, a board does not really exist unless it is meeting. Consequently, maximizing use of this precious time is the essence of the art of good governance. An effective board controls how it spends its meeting time; an ineffective board does not. How does a board control its members' time together? By controlling its meeting agenda and the information it receives.

By developing the strategic plan and the annual organizational goals and objectives, and by refining these into annual board goals and objectives, the board has already identified the critical issues it should be spending its time on. The next step is to translate these issues into agenda items and to have the discipline to stick to them.

Many boards become prisoners of their own agendas. Their meetings seem to be structured so that the most meaningless, mundane, small-picture issues come first on the agenda and consume most of the meeting time. Significant big-picture issues, if addressed at all, often are placed at the end of the agenda, when the board either feels time pressure to end the meeting or runs out of time or energy to adequately address them. Often,

> ... the board agenda is not the *board's* agenda but administration's agenda for the board. Board meetings are more a matter of hearing reports than of struggling with and resolving momentous issues.[2]

For a board agenda to truly be the *board's* agenda, it must flow from the goals and objectives developed by and for the board. Consistent with board goals and objectives, the most important items to be discussed should be placed at the beginning of the agenda. This ensures that a board will in fact address the most important issues confronting the organization or system. How will board members know what the most important issues are? They will already have determined that in the earlier steps of the effective governance pyramid process.

The significant issues found in the strategic plan, the organizational goals and objectives, the annual board goals and objectives, and the board committee work plans form the critical agenda issues for the board. If the board can identify the critical issues confronting the system or organization (as it has done in the earlier steps of the pyramid), it will have structured its own agenda for the year.

Boards that do not do this find that their agenda is opportunistic and situational. Whatever situation that arises assumes an air of great importance, not because it *is* important but, rather, because the board does not have a collective sense of what is important. This type of board spends its time on whatever is happening, and its members persuade themselves that their meetings are meaningful when, in fact, members are at best spending all their time "putting out fires" or spinning their wheels.

A sense of purpose and priority is critical for a board to function with consistent effectiveness. This purpose and priority must be reflected in the board's agenda. Effective boards demonstrate a rigorous agenda control and the discipline to stick to the agenda.

A useful technique being used by a growing number of boards to address necessary, legally required, or other small-picture issues (such as approval of minutes, receipt of routine reports, and so on) is the consent agenda. In the consent agenda, routine items are grouped together under one agenda item, and relevant materials are included under one section of the board agenda book. Board members read this section prior to coming to the meeting, and if no one has any questions or concerns, the entire block of issues is accepted or approved with one board vote and no discussion. This frees up a significant amount of meeting time that would otherwise be wasted on ceremonial, legal, or parliamentary procedure.

In addition to using the consent agenda, effective boards organize their agendas for action. An action agenda can be structured as follows:

A. Action items
   1. Consent (routine) items
   2. Substantive items
B. Discussion items
C. Information items
D. Open-agenda items

The action agenda is organized so that items requiring immediate board action are addressed first. These are followed by items requiring board discussion and deliberation.

The discussion items at the current board meeting are likely to be the action items at a subsequent meeting. This is an important point because effective boards strive to build a culture of performance and accountability where members support development of the board as a group, focus on the collective welfare of the board, and develop a sense of group cohesiveness. One way to accomplish this is to rarely have a vote on a major issue at the meeting in which it is first presented to the board. Effective boards encourage discussion of issues among their members and do not rush their decision making. The action agenda facilitates group cohesion and effective decision making by encouraging discussion and deliberation on an issue at one meeting, and then bringing that issue up for a decision at a subsequent meeting. This approach encourages deliberation and also foreshadows future decision points.

Board Information Control

There are three general types of information in a system or health care organization: management, clinical, and governance. If a board is given management information, it will manage. If a board is given clinical information, it will attempt to practice medicine.

Boards respond to the information they are provided. This is why it is critical to provide boards with governance information. Unfortunately, many boards do not receive governance information in their agenda materials. Rather, they get operational detail, warmed-over management reports, and detailed clinical information.

Following are common flaws and weaknesses in providing information and reports to boards:

- Reports and information do not flow from or support the explicitly defined role of the board regarding the issue.

- There are no guidelines on what information should be reported to the board or how it should be reported.
- Reports provide data (such as cross-sectional indicators) but not information (such as longitudinal trends or projections).
- Meeting minutes are used as the primary vehicle for providing information to the board (for example, the finance committee minutes are used as the financial report to the board).
- Too much material is presented in the reports.
- Ineffective report formats blunt the board's understanding of important information.

To avoid these flaws, information provided to the board should be brief and in graphic format whenever possible. Any narratives provided to the board should be prefaced by an executive summary. The information provided should relate directly to the strategy, the organizational goals, and the annual board goals and objectives. Finally, meeting minutes should never be used as the primary vehicle for providing information to the board.

If information provided the board reflects an issue that has been considered by another group in the organization subordinate to the board (such as a board or management committee), the board should receive a summary distillation of the information the group below considered. Figure 4-2 offers a graphic example of this point. Imagine that a system

Figure 4-2. Effective Governance Information Flow

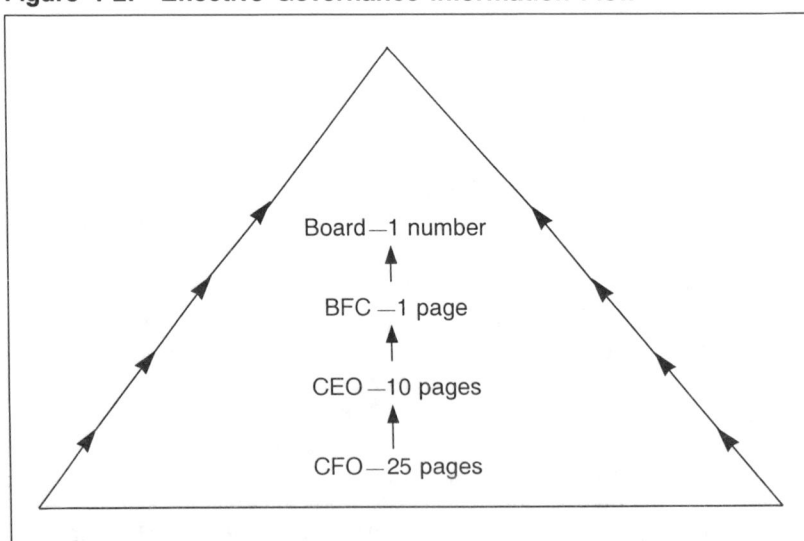

©Copyright 1996, Orlikoff & Associates, Chicago.

chief financial officer (CFO) is addressing a particular issue, such as days cash on hand. The CFO might consider 25 pages of information on this issue. Now, the CEO probably also considers this same issue. If both the CEO and the CFO consider the same issue, what, then, is the difference in their jobs? The difference is authority and oversight, and level of detail reviewed. Thus, the CEO might only see 10 pages of information on days cash on hand. Next, a report on this issue is made to the Board Finance Committee (BFC). If the BFC sees 25 pages of information on the subject, the committee will in effect be doing the CFO's job. Thus, the BFC might only see one page of information on days cash on hand. This same issue also might be reported to the board, but the board might only be provided with one number, along with target points or upper- and lower-control limits.

In this way, the board can exercise appropriate oversight without duplicating the information review conducted by the groups or individuals below it. Of course, should the one number or indicator received by the board be outside the target range or control limits, the board could ask for more information. This "drilling down" for information is only done by the board when the governance indicators warrant it. (To complete the example, suppose the board had determined that it did not want the system's days cash on hand to fall below 15 or to rise above 50. In the event the one number the board receives is above or below those limits, the board could drill down for more information to determine the reason for the trend and the action to correct it.)

Unfortunately, many boards do not follow this process. Ineffective boards follow a process graphically depicted in figure 4-3. However, this is not the worst example of governance information flow. That honor is depicted in figure 4-4. In figure 4-4, the board is actually seeing more data than the groups below it need to do their jobs. This type of governance is not only ineffective, it is dysfunctional.

Related Governance Issues

The effective governance pyramid also provides the basis for many other key governance activities. The annual board goals and objectives should provide the foundation for the board education and retreat process. Additionally, they should become criteria for the new board member recruitment process and the basis for the new board member orientation process.

As an example, again imagine that an organization has the strategy of merging with another entity to facilitate an IDS formation. A board goal and objective is to facilitate such a merger. In addition to assigning specific tasks to the board committees as described earlier, the board also can use this as a criterion for selecting new members. Specifically, the

Figure 4-3. Ineffective Governance Information Flow

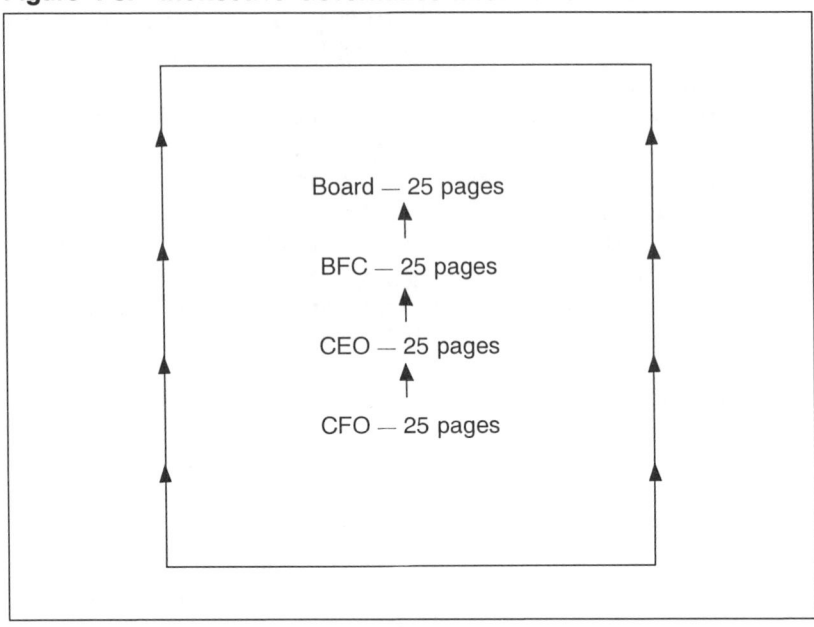

©Copyright 1996, Orlikoff & Associates, Chicago.

Figure 4-4. Dysfunctional Governance Information Flow

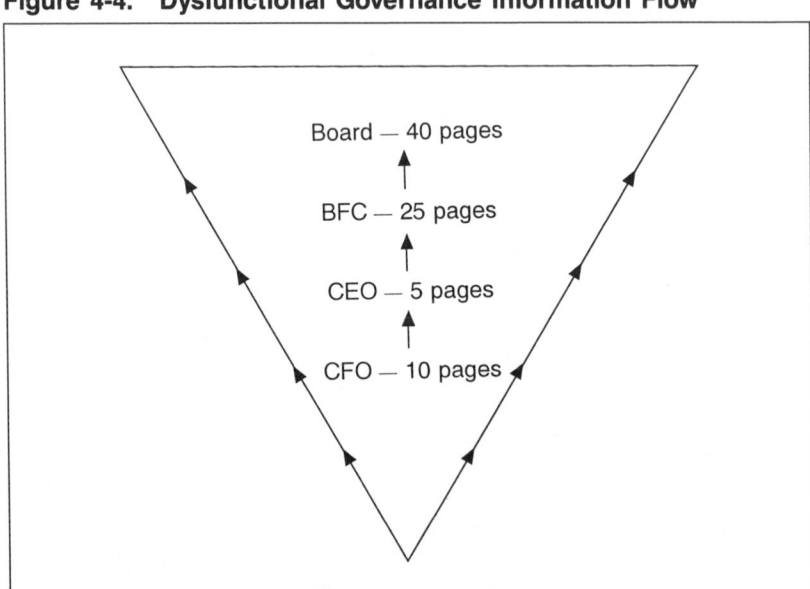

©Copyright 1996, Orlikoff & Associates, Chicago.

board might choose to seek a businessperson who has had experience with mergers, an attorney who specializes in mergers and affiliations, or an organizational psychologist who concentrates in efficiently blending different organizational cultures in a postmerger environment.

Thus, the base of the effective governance pyramid affects every board function and structure, including composition, new member recruitment and orientation, and education.

Evaluation

The one activity that ties the effective governance pyramid together is evaluation. The annual board goals and objectives form the basis for the annual board self-evaluation. The CEO performance objectives form the basis for the CEO performance evaluation. Just as the board and CEO objectives should be developed in tandem, so should the two evaluation processes be conducted together. This emphasizes the leadership continuum between governance and management—the interdependency that effective governance and management share.

A well-constructed CEO performance evaluation and board self-evaluation process can help both board members and management improve their performance and achieve and maintain excellence in governance and management. Self-evaluation provides a board with a structured opportunity to both look back and plan ahead. The process allows the board to ask itself questions such as:

- What are we doing well?
- What could we be doing better?
- What are our objectives?
- How well did we achieve our objectives?
- Why did we not achieve our objectives?

The board then uses the answers to these questions to develop an action plan to improve its performance and establish new goals.

Conclusion of the two evaluation processes leads into the next cycle of the effective governance pyramid, and the process begins again for the coming year. Specifically, the process begins again at the base of the pyramid with the review and reaffirmation or revision of the mission, the refinement of the strategic plan or development of new strategies, and so on.

Vision

The object of the effective governance pyramid is twofold: to achieve the mission, and to accomplish the vision. The mission, discussed earlier, is what the system or organization is. The vision is what the board wishes the system to become at some point in the future. By framing the effective governance pyramid between the mission and the vision, the board establishes a dynamic, creative tension. It is through this tension that board members formulate effective policy, make meaningful decisions, and lead their system into the future. Additionally, it is through this tension that the board is able to transform itself.

A Practical Tip for Maintaining Focus

The effective governance pyramid enables a board to remain focused, conduct mini-evaluations throughout the year, and perform midcourse corrections. However, to truly benefit, the board must follow the effective governance pyramid.

A practical and easy way to do this is to place the pyramid, or its key parts, in front of the board and its committees at each meeting. For example, for the board, the first page of each agenda book should include the base of the pyramid—the mission and the key strategic goals. The second page should list the annual board goals and objectives. For board committees, the first page of each agenda book likewise should include the mission and the key strategic goals, but the second page should show the annual committee work plan.

Through this simple technique, the priorities, focus, and purpose of the board and its committees are clear to all the members of the different governance entities. Further, each member can help keep the board on track by questioning discussion that is not relevant to the base of the effective governance pyramid.

As a practical example of this technique, consider Wesley Woods, Inc., an Atlanta-based integrated system of geriatric and long-term care. It includes a 100-bed geriatric hospital with an outpatient clinic; 340 nursing home beds; outpatient primary care and specialty assessment and treatment services; a comprehensive outpatient rehabilitation facility; seven residential retirement living facilities; and biomedical research facilities.

How does the Wesley Woods board stay on top of this system and focused on its key strategies? The answer is through its own version of the effective governance pyramid. Figure 4-5 (pp. 58–59) shows the Wesley Woods Vision Alignment Matrix® (VAM) for 1995–1997. Notice that it contains most of the elements of the effective governance pyramid: mission, vision, strategies, and tactics. The VAM appears on the first page of every agenda book at every Wesley Woods board meeting.

The Governance Committee

Many boards find it useful to assign responsibility for implementation of the effective governance pyramid to a board committee, as opposed to carving up the tasks among different committees. For example, rather than relying on their traditional nominating committee, many boards rely on a governance committee (sometimes called the *Board Development Committee*). The purpose of this committee is to assist the board in fulfilling its ultimate responsibility for ensuring its own effective and efficient performance—in other words, to assist the board in the construction and implementation of the effective governance pyramid.

Typical functions of the governance committee include:

- Formulating draft annual board goals and objectives
- Suggesting annual committee structure and annual board committee work plans
- Planning board education, including new trustee orientation and board retreats
- Effecting new board member identification and recruitment
- Evaluating trustee performance pursuant to reappointment to additional terms of office
- Nominating board officers
- Effecting board self-evaluation

Thus, the functions of the governance committee include the nominations process but go far beyond that to present an integrated approach to facilitating excellence in governance.

Conclusion

Effective governance is not a happy accident. Rather, it is the result of an integrated process of planning, coordination, implementation, and evaluation. By following tradition or simply responding to whatever situations arise, governance abdicates its responsibility for leadership and contributes to organizational atrophy. Although effective governance is more art than science, it can be achieved through a structured process such as the effective governance pyramid.

References

1. Chait, R. P., and Taylor, B. E. Charting the territory of nonprofit boards. *Harvard Business Review,* Jan.–Feb. 1989, p. 54.
2. Carver, J. To focus on shaping the future, many hospital boards might require a radical overhaul. *The Baxter Foundation's Health Management Quarterly* 16(1):7, First Quarter 1994.

Figure 4-5. Wesley Woods, Inc., Vision Alignment Matrix® (1995–1997)

	Strategies:		
Mission Statement To help people age in healthy, affordable, and ethical ways through service, education, and research.	Develop Wesley Woods' role in the Emory System of Healthcare. **1**	Excel in customer satisfaction and quality of care. **2**	Develop a chronic care network as part of an integrated delivery system. **3**
Values Statement Compassion, respect, commitment, competency, collaboration, innovation, stewardship, and inclusiveness.	**Tactics:**		
	1-1 (Red): Redefine master relationship agreement with Emory.	2-1 (Red): Improve customer satisfaction feedback and response mechanism.	3-1 (Red): Define the assessment program.
Vision Statement Wesley Woods, Inc. will be the preeminent comprehensive geriatric center in the nation by the year 2000.	1-2 (Red): Formalize administrative and planning relationship.	2-2 (Red): Cultivate employee's understanding of the corporate mission and vision.	3-2 (Red): Implement A. G. Rhodes relationship.
	1-3 (Red): Refine the acute and primary care service.	2-3 (Red): Implement customer relations training programs around CQI principles.	3-3 (Red): Implement "case management" service/system.
Customers Donors, employees, families, patients, payers, physicians, providers, residents, suppliers, volunteers, Emory University of Healthcare and the North Georgia Annual Conference of the United Methodist Church.	1-4 (Red): Develop a concerted long-term care service.	2-4 (Red): Develop a long-range parking and transportation plan.	3-4 (Red): Develop a concerted affiliate network.
	1-5 (Red): Develop a concerted rehab service.	2-5 (Orange): Standardize corporate image, materials, and signage.	3-5 (Orange): Redefine the LTCH program.
	1-6 (Red): Refine academic plan.	2-6 (Green): Renovate facilities as necessary to meet new markets.	3-6 (Orange): Redefine support services/programs in residential facilities (assisted living).
	1-7 (Orange): Develop a concerted home health service.	2-7 (Green): Achieve and maintain JCAHO and EAGLE accreditation.	3-7 (Orange): Develop managed care approach to service through demonstration grant approach.
Philosophy Statement Consistent with Judeo-Christian values, we believe aging has a fulfilling purpose in life. Further, we believe society is strong to the extent that elders are valued, the organization is strong to the extent people and resources are respected; and the organization is worthy of community support to the extent it provides exemplary public service.	1-8 (Orange): Expand ECT.	2-8	3-8 (Orange): Begin construction in current and new markets areas (Athens, Newnan).
	1-9 (Orange): Develop partial hospital program.	2-9	3-9 (Orange): Implement PACE program.
	1-10 (Orange): Determine feasibility of substance abuse program.	2-10	3-10
	1-11 (Orange): Develop academic nursing shared vision/program.	2-11	3-11
	1-12 (Yellow): Develop residential program role in the Emory System.	2-12	3-12

Legend: Red = Crucial to survival; Orange = Accomplish in 1996; Yellow = Accomplish in 1997; Green = Ongoing

Reprinted, with permission, from William L. Minnix, Jr., president and CEO, Wesley Woods Geriatric Hospital, Inc., Atlanta. The term *Vision Alignment Matrix* is registered by, and the Vision Alignment Process was developed by, Avatar International Inc. They can be reached at 1-800-AVATAR4.

A Framework for Effective Governance

Reinforce a healthy, educated, productive, diverse, paid and volunteer staff. 4	Achieve and maintain financial viability. 5	Redefine the research and education plan and integrate into services. 6	Redefine and implement a structure to carry out the programs of the organization. 7
4-1 (Red): Refine continuous quality improvement team work.	5-1 (Red): Achieve financial budgets (plans)	6-1 (Red): Achieve and maintain research program viability.	7-1 (Red): Provide for systems support to address program needs.
4-2 (Red): Implement performance and compensation plan.	5-2 (Red): Fund depreciation at target percentage of annual depreciation expense.	6-2 (Red): Develop business plan and implementation schedule for neuroscience program.	7-2 (Red): Implement information systems improvement plan.
4-3 (Orange): Develop and implement a new volunteer plan.	5-3 (Red): Implement major capital and endowment campaign.	6-3 (Orange): Target corporate foundation plans for research initiatives.	7-3 (Red): Organize and deliver care around structured models.
4-4 (Orange): Redefine employee benefits program.	5-4 (Red): Develop contingency plans based on public policy changes.	6-4	7-4 (Red): Revise marketing and strategic managing processes.
4-5 (Green): Utilize the strengths of the organization's diverse work force.	5-5 (Orange): Develop a capital budget.	6-5	7-5 (Red): Refine business planning process.
4-6 (Green): Refine education plan for staff, volunteers, and customers.	5-6 (Green): Develop marketing plans to achieve revenue objectives.	6-6	7-6 (Orange): Redefine corporate structure to facilitate affiliate network.
4-7	5-7 (Green): Evaluate financial arrangements with affiliates.	6-7	7-7 (Orange): Develop a board education and development plan.
4-8	5-8 (Green): Explore alternative revenue sources.	6-8	7-8
4-9	5-9	6-9	7-9
4-10	5-10	6-10	7-10
4-11	5-11	6-11	7-11
4-12	5-12	6-12	7-12

Chapter 5

A Process for Restructuring Governance

The term *governance restructuring* encompasses many things—reducing the number of board members, changing a board's committee structure, restructuring the number and function of boards in an established integrated delivery system (IDS), creating the governance function and structure of a newly forming IDS, and so on. This chapter addresses several key issues and methods involved in conducting a governance restructuring process.

Governance Structure and Function Revisited

It is useful to begin by repeating a caveat mentioned in chapter 4—that form should follow function. A process that simply focuses on changing or streamlining the structure of governance without first addressing its function (especially the relative roles and responsibilities of multiple boards) is likely to cause more problems than it solves. Although it is typical to revise governance function at the same time that structure is addressed, many governance redesign efforts focus only on structural issues.

The temptation to address structural issues alone exists because the structure of governance is more tangible than its function. Addressing how many board committees there should be is easier than talking about what the board should do and how its work should be organized. Yet, before issues such as number of board members, number or type of board committees, or number and type of boards in a system can be determined intelligently, the functions of the board(s) must be clear.

For example, suppose a hospital determines that one of its board's key roles is to be a vehicle for involving community members. In this case, a key function of the board necessitates a certain structural characteristic—namely, that the board will have a large number of members. This functional choice will have other structural ramifications as well. If the board is in fact very large (over 30 members), it will most likely need an executive committee that is invested with authority to take broad and frequent action without seeking board approval. Further, to provide avenues for adequate levels of input for all the many board members, it is likely that the board will have a large number of board committees.

Now assume that due to a cumbersome decision-making process, an excessive consumption of chief executive officer (CEO) time, and an unfocused board–committee relationship, the hospital CEO and the board chair express the need to reduce the board's size and streamline the number of its committees. This can be done with relative ease but will result in fewer opportunities for community members to directly participate in the governance of the institution. Here, the structural revision will inhibit one of the board's key functions.

In this example, as in most governance situations, a delicate latticework of interrelated factors, both structural and functional, exists. To change one of the variables in the belief that the others will not be affected is naive. To change one of the variables without thinking through the whole process—the whole gestalt—of governance is usually deleterious to both governance and the system or organization being governed.

Thus, governance structure and function are inexorably intertwined, and so should be considered together in any governance redesign or restructuring process. Structure cannot be dismissed as unimportant because it provides:

> . . . the channels and safeguards for productive thought and action. Only as a board is freed to carry out its functions with vigor and imagination is it infused with life. . . . "The flour is the important thing, not the mill." And yet, you cannot have the flour without the mill. . . .[1]

Basic Steps for Governance Redesign

A governance redesign process should be composed of several basic steps, including:

1. Form a governance committee or task force to develop recommendations for restructuring the governance of an IDS or organization (or assign this task to a standing group).
2. Develop conceptual governance principles and redesign goals.
3. Evaluate the current health care organization or IDS governance structure in relation to these principles.
4. Develop specific recommendations to restructure the governance of the system or organization.
5. Approve and implement the recommendations.

Each of these steps is discussed in the following subsections, pp. 64–69.

Form a Governance Redesign Task Force

Frequently, an organization or system will call in an outside consultant to conduct a governance restructuring process. Although content expertise is indeed valuable to the process, the greatest value and best outcomes are achieved through a consensus-based approach to developing recommendations to restructure and improve the governance function and process.

To have the greatest value, and to maintain the mission touchstones of the system, the recommendations should come from an internal group, not an external consultant. This means that in addition to content expertise and advice, a consultant should provide facilitation expertise.

Working with an entire board on the details and logistics of a governance restructuring process is usually too cumbersome or politically charged to be conducted successfully. Thus, it is better to have a task force, a special committee, or a governance design team address the issues relating to the redesign process.

An outside expert can help facilitate task force or special committee consideration, consensus, and recommendations on redesigning the governance process and structure for a health care organization or system. The task force or special committee should include members from existing governance structures in the system, as well as key current and future stakeholders of the system. Further, this group should be given a specific charge and timetable.

This is not to say that the organization's existing governance entity will not be involved in the process. Indeed, the process cannot proceed to implementation without the approval of one or several governance entities. For this reason, it is advisable to involve the relevant governing board(s) at specific points throughout the process.

An initial board retreat is a useful beginning to a restructuring project for several reasons. First, it establishes the need as well as sets the stage for governance restructuring. Second, it provides board, management, and physician leadership with a foreshadowing of the issues involved and the likely direction of the project. Third, it helps the outside consultant assess the dynamics of the interaction among board members, executive staff, and physician leadership.

In a governance restructuring process conducted in a system with multiple boards, it is important to build in a "check-in" process with the other boards. This enables the boards to ensure that the direction of the special committee or task force is both appropriate and politically acceptable.

Often the process will culminate with another board retreat to present, discuss, and approve the recommendations of the governance redesign task force and to achieve board approval for, and commitment to, implementation of the restructuring plan. Depending on the nature of the recommendations, this also can be done at a regularly scheduled meeting of the board(s).

Develop Conceptual Principles and Goals

Once the governance restructuring special committee or task force is formed, its first task should be to develop a set of conceptual governance principles. These will be the guiding principles for the governance structure redesign and so must be conceptual enough to provide flexibility, but specific enough to provide direction to the task force.

It is through these governance principles that the values, history, culture, beliefs, and traditions of the system (or of several organizations coming together to form a system) will be maintained. Absent such principles, the essence or culture of a system or organization will likely be lost or rendered unrecognizable in the governance redesign process.

Following are actual examples of conceptual principles and goals for governance restructuring from a variety of organizations and systems that have gone through the process:

- Governance decision-making processes must be streamlined, and the cycle time of decision making must be reduced as much as possible.
- The governance structure and function will support the mission of the system.
- The governance structure will support the IDS strategy.
- The governance structure and function should further the financial health of the organization.
- The goals of streamlining governance structure (reducing the number of boards) and maintaining community involvement in governance must be balanced.
- Multiple boards are a critical component of our commitment to involve as many community members and system stakeholders as possible in the governance of our IDS. Therefore, this process should not result in a reduction of the number of boards or board members. It will focus on improving the function of the boards and the overall quality of governance of the system by: improving the information flow between the boards and other leadership groups; clarifying the relative roles and responsibilities of the different governance entities; clearly delineating the reserved powers and decision-

making authority of the system board; and streamlining and integrating the committee structures of the boards.
- The board should be reduced in size, with term limits imposed, while maintaining board continuity during trustee turnover.
- The members of the system board (of an IDS) should be largely, but not exclusively, drawn from the pool of board members of the subordinate organizations within the system. However, under no circumstances will any subordinate organization be guaranteed "slots" on the system board.
- The redesigned structure of system governance must be flexible enough to integrate all future partnerships, affiliations, and acquisitions to facilitate the formation of an IDS.
- The parent corporation must be not-for-profit but can have for-profit subsidiary organizations.
- The governance structure will be as streamlined as possible, with a system board and as few subsidiary boards as possible.
- The governance structures must provide significant opportunities for physician involvement and membership on boards and their committees.
- A majority of system board members shall be members of the sponsoring religious order.
- Executive management time devoted to governance activities should represent no more than 25 percent of total executive management time.
- Time demands on board members who are not officers or committee chairs should not exceed an average of 20 hours per month.
- A better use of board member expertise and experience; retain the philanthropic fund-raising potential of board members while reducing the size of the parent board; streamline and focus the work of the board committees.

Whether the conceptual principles are general or specific, they should be a projection of the most important values of the system's leadership. These principles are expressions of what is to be preserved as well as what is to be created during the process of change. Absent such principles, it is very possible to design a new governance structure and process that eliminates all the positive structural and functional aspects from the past governance process while adding nothing new of value.

Once the special committee or task force develops a draft of the conceptual principles for governance redesign, the draft should be submitted to the board(s) for buy-in and approval. This helps involve the entire board(s) in the process, as well as commits the board to accept the committee's final specific recommendations, if they are indeed consistent with the conceptual governance principles.

Evaluate the Current Function and Structure

After the conceptual principles have been developed and approved, the current governance function and structure should be assessed. This phase involves the comparison and evaluation of all aspects of the current system or organization's governance structure and function against the established governance principles. This serves to identify the specific areas and activities in need of change, as well as those that should be retained.

During this phase of the process, one useful technique is to have the CEO assess how much CEO and senior executive management time is spent on governance functions. This technique includes assessing the time spent on preparing for board meetings; attending board and board committee meetings; writing minutes; speaking with trustees after the meetings regarding the process and conclusions of the meetings; and planning and attending board retreats and education conferences.

According to research conducted by The Governance Institute, there is wide variation in the amount of time CEOs spend on governance-related work. For both hospital and system CEOs, the research found that about 39 percent spend 10 hours or less a month on governance, 38 percent spend between 11 and 20 hours a month, 10 percent spend between 21 and 30 hours a month, and 12 percent spend 31 or more hours a month.[2] An assessment of CEO and senior executive time spent on governance could result in development of an additional governance principle relating to the maximum amount of time CEOs should spend on governance.

Similarly, it would be useful to have board members assess how much time they devote to governance. An average time commitment per month, as well as an overall range of time spent, could yield interesting information and suggest avenues of meaningful restructuring.

Following is an example of the results of an actual governance evaluation of a system:

- Our system board is too large to make quick decisions in a rapidly changing market.
- We have far too many subordinate boards, which consume too much of executive management's time and waste the time of board members who serve on several of the boards and hear the same reports over and over.
- There is dangerous confusion over relative roles and authority among different subsidiary boards in the system, and especially between the [major medical center] board and the system board. This creates the great probability of conflict or gridlock between these two governance entities in the near future.

- The lack of term limits has created an inbred system board that is lacking in drive and innovation. There is a great reluctance to remove nonperforming board members.
- The system board is locked into the hospital paradigm and is not really functioning as a system board; rather, it is a glorified hospital board. The system board does not truly understand the changing health care environment, and this is reflected in its function and its committee structure.

Develop Specific Recommendations

The next step in this process is to facilitate specific recommendations to restructure and improve the governance process of the system or organization. These recommendations would flow from both the conceptual governance principles and the evaluation of the strengths and weaknesses of the current governance structure and function.

As a result of the preceding three steps, the recommendations developed will reflect the specific needs and circumstances of the individual system or organization, as opposed to being an off-the-shelf series of recommendations. Once the conceptual governance principles have been established and the governance assessment conducted, the specific recommendations to restructure governance are often self-evident. (An example of a set of recommendations to restructure governance is presented in a case study at the end of chapter 6.)

Approve and Implement the Recommendations

The final phase of the process involves presenting the governance redesign task force's recommendations for formal approval to the system board or, in the case of several organizations merging to create a system, to the various organizational boards. As indicated earlier, often this is best done at a board retreat so that board members can question and debate the recommendations and consider their implications in depth.

This is a crucial event because it is at this point in the governance redesign process that those board members not on the governance redesign task force will truly begin to understand, at an emotional level, the scope of the recommended changes. They will begin to realize how the changes will affect either them personally or the components of the system they are most invested in. For example, the changes frequently will involve many of the board members being excluded from the newly formed governance entities. Further, the changes may involve the actual or apparent diminution of the boards of certain organizations that once were the powerhouses or cash cows of the system. The changes also may involve a new form of, or approach to, governance that is radically different from that of the past (for example, compensating board members, moving away from a community representative board, changing the board selection process, and so on).

Such changes do not come without challenge. Several board members may not be able to abide the changes, and will vehemently argue against them and possibly resign from the board if the changes are approved. This is an expected and acceptable occurrence. It is critically important to accept that it is very difficult to radically change the governance process and keep all past board members involved in it.

In addition to providing a forum in which these feelings can be vented, the board retreat offers an opportunity to celebrate the past governance process and recognize those who participated in it. It must be emphasized that the past governance process was not bad and its participants were not wrong for having been part of it, but that times have changed and new times call for new governance.

Once the governance redesign recommendations are approved by the board, the next step is to actually implement them. Although this may seem to be the greatest challenge, it often is less difficult than gaining board approval to implement recommendations that may represent significant change.

As a result of a governance restructuring process, some boards may be asked to vote themselves out of existence, some may be asked to accept an advisory role to a new governance entity, and some may be asked to have all their members voluntarily resign so that the board can be reconstituted with new members. These are perhaps the most difficult decisions for a board to make. That is why it is critical to follow the consensus-based process outlined in this chapter.

By doing so, the final recommendations are foreshadowed by the process, and gradually the board members buy in one step at a time. This is why it is crucial to include board members on the governance redesign team and to have several check-in points with the board as a whole at the conclusion of each phase of the process (for example, after development of the governance principles, after evaluation of the current governance structure, and after preliminary development of the restructuring recommendations). Thus, once developed, the final recommendations are not a surprise and, in fact, have an air of inevitability about them. If the process outlined in this chapter is followed, it will be extremely rare that a board will reject or even significantly modify the governance redesign recommendations put before it.

The entire process takes, on average, about six months to one year. However, it can be accelerated with more frequent meetings or if the governance redesign committee moves through its work quickly. It also is possible that it may take longer depending on the dynamics of the redesign committee and the receptiveness of the boards to the committee's recommendations.

Conclusion

This chapter's approach to a governance restructuring project will result in development of specific, detailed recommendations that logically interrelate to improve the governance function, structure, relationships, and information flow. The final result usually represents a total approach that restructures and improves the system of governance, as opposed to a piecemeal approach that tweaks some of its parts.

References

1. Houle, C. O. *Governing Boards: Their Nature and Nurture.* San Francisco: Jossey-Bass, 1989, p. 84.
2. The Governance Institute. *Governance Trends and Practices in Health Systems: 1995 Panel Survey of System Boards.* La Jolla, CA: The Governance Institute, 1995.

Chapter 6

Issues in System Governance Structure

Governance structure does not determine governance function; rather, it can only facilitate or inhibit effective governance function. As mentioned earlier, there is little agreement on the ideal governance structure for an integrated delivery system (IDS) for a very good reason: The structure for the governance of each system should be determined primarily by the unique and individually defined needs, culture, and mission of each system.

Nevertheless, as a health care organization or system moves toward a revision of its governance process, several critical issues regarding the structure of the new governance entity must be addressed. For example:

- Should the system have centralized or decentralized governance?
- If decentralized governance is chosen, should the system have governance structures divided by region, function, or specific organization?
- How should board member selection be performed?
- Should the board be representational or self-perpetuating?
- What should the size of the board(s) be?
- Should board members be compensated?
- How should physician involvement in governance be structured?
- Should board member terms of office be limited?
- Should the IDS corporate parent be a not-for-profit entity?

Within the context of the process for redesigning governance presented in chapter 5, these and other questions are addressed in the development of conceptual governance principles, the evaluation of the current governance structure, and the development of specific recommendations. This chapter discusses several of these issues and examines the advantages and disadvantages of each option. The chapter concludes with a case study of an IDS that restructured its governance forms and functions.

Should Governance Be Centralized or Decentralized?

Some integrated delivery systems (IDSs) are moving toward a single corporate board, which is a centralized governance approach. Others have multiple layers of boards and share authority and function among them, which is called decentralized governance. Some IDSs choose to have a single parent board with advisory boards for each organization, but the majority of IDSs currently employ some type of multiple-board, decentralized governance approach.

In a centralized governance structure, a single board with ultimate authority and reserved power directly oversees all system components, with either no other boards or "advisory" boards only. In a decentralized governance structure, the system board oversees or coordinates several subordinate boards. A compromise between the two is a "modified centralized" governance structure, with a parent system board and as few subsidiary boards as possible (usually three or fewer).

Centralized Governance Structure

The advantages of a single-board or centralized governance structure with severely streamlined boards are:

- Consolidation of oversight and control into one or as few governance entities as possible
- Facilitation of rapid governance decision making
- Minimization of executive management time required to staff and support governance functions
- An increased tendency for the board to place the interests of the system as a whole above the interests of any of its component parts
- An increased tendency for the board to focus on policy and planning, rather than operations, due to system size and complexity

The disadvantages of this governance structure are:

- Restriction on the number of community members and other IDS stakeholders who can participate in the governance of the system
- The risk that the board may become too far removed from oversight of the system
- Rapid governance decision making without input from key IDS stakeholders
- A loss of system marketing effectiveness due to the loss of several board members who may have been influential in the community

Decentralized Governance Structure

It is a unique characteristic of multihospital systems and IDSs that they have multiple or tiered governance structures.[1] These multiple boards exist within the same organization and have superior–subordinate relationships.

The advantages of a decentralized governance structure with multiple boards are:

- It provides the opportunity to push selected board responsibilities and functions down to the level where they can be fulfilled with greater sensitivity to the distinctive circumstances faced by the various components of the system.
- Due to a greater number of boards, there is the opportunity to involve a large number of community members and other IDS stakeholders in governance of the system.
- Multiple boards can accomplish greater volumes of governance work and can conduct more detailed system component oversight and monitoring because the governance functions can be divided among the different boards.
- Responsibilities of the individual boards can be prescribed to focus the work of each individual board.

The disadvantages of this governance structure are:

- Governance ineffectiveness due to more cumbersome decision-making processes and diffusion of each board's focus and commitment. Proposals and reports must be reviewed at several levels, so decision-making time is increased.
- Difficulty in coordinating work and integrated decision making; potential for "governance gridlock."
- Potential for conflict between the boards regarding relative authority and responsibility or regarding allocation or use of system resources.
- Different boards being prone to representational governance; that is, being likely to represent the interests of "their" component part as opposed to the interests of the system as a whole, impeding system performance and advancement.
- Multiple boards placing inordinate time and energy demands on executive management who must staff and support each of the boards. This detracts from effective system management and operation.

How Should Decentralized Governance Functions Be Divided?

If an IDS pursues decentralized governance, governance functions must be subdivided among the multiple layers of boards. The question becomes: How should the functions and responsibilities of governance be defined, performed, and coordinated among the different boards?

There are three ways to do this.[2] The governance divisions can be *regional*, where boards subordinate to the system board are created for each geographic market or region where the system operates; *functional*, where subordinate boards are created to oversee groupings of system components that perform similar functions (such as hospitals, physician groups, insurance entities, and so on); or *organizational*, where each component organization of the system is overseen by a subordinate board. The advantages and disadvantages of these three approaches are very similar.

Regional Governance Divisions

The advantages of regional governance divisions are:

- A minimal number of boards in a decentralized governance structure
- Community members and other system stakeholders being involved in the governance of the system specific to their region
- System board concentration on planning for the whole system and coordination among the regional areas

The disadvantages of regional governance divisions are:

- Tendency for regional representational governance
- Artificial distinctions between regions that can inhibit the system's ability to function smoothly across regional lines
- Facilitation of regional variation in operation, quality, and cost efficiency, which is diametrically opposed to the concept of systemness

Functional Governance Divisions

Although an IDS could have an infinite variety of functional governance distinctions, there are three that are basic: insurance functions, physician functions, and care delivery functions.

The advantages of functional governance divisions are:

- Each subordinate governance entity concentrates exclusively on oversight of a specific functional area (such as hospitals, physician

groups, nursing homes, and so on), which can bring a clear focus to governance function within an IDS.
- Community members and stakeholders can be involved in the governance of the system, but in their specific areas of interest.
- The system board concentrates on planning for the whole system and coordination among the functional areas.
- It may be easier to recruit board members with desired specific expertise and interest to a board with a more specific functional focus.

The disadvantages of functional governance divisions are:

- Governance can tend to become representational of specific functions.
- Smooth systems operation and oversight across the continuum of different functions may be inhibited.
- Different functional groups may develop different corporate and operational cultures inconsistent with the direction envisioned by the system board.

Organizational Governance Divisions

The advantages of organizational governance divisions are:

- Community and stakeholder involvement in governance can be maximized due to the large number of boards; one board for each organization.
- Each subordinate governance entity concentrates on oversight of a single organization.

The disadvantages of organizational governance divisions are:

- Highest risk of governance gridlock, as well as conflict among boards due to their large number and each having a narrow focus.
- Greatest demand on executive management time as all boards will need to be staffed, prepared for, communicated with, and functionally and strategically coordinated.
- Encouragement of representational governance as each board is charged with oversight of a specific organization. If the system board is composed of representatives of the subordinate boards, the representative emphasis will inhibit effective system governance.

How Should Board Member Selection Be Performed?

Once the determination is made regarding the type of governance model to implement and the number of boards to have, the issue of how to select board members must be addressed. There are three basic approaches to selecting system and subordinate board members: the elected board, the appointed board, and the self-perpetuating board.

The Elected Board

The elected board is one where members are actually elected by either people in a particular geographic area or the members of a particular constituent or economic group.

The advantages of the elected board model are:

- Community involvement in the selection process
- The potential for board accountability directly to the public
- The potential for board representation of public interests

The disadvantages of elected boards are:

- Elected boards frequently become political and are less likely to understand their role in relation to management and systems thinking.
- Elected boards usually have extremely limited trustee terms, so there is frequent trustee turnover that contributes to sporadic and ineffective board function.
- Continuity of board function is inhibited.
- Individuals with specific agendas may campaign for office and, upon election to the board, focus only on their specific area of interest to the exclusion and detriment of their many other governance functions and responsibilities.
- The board can exercise no control over dysfunctional members because the power to remove members rests with the electorate.
- Self-evaluation tends to be ineffective in improving board performance.

The Appointed Board

In the appointed board, members are selected and appointed to office by either a governmental or religious body, or an individual with elected or corporate authority. Typical groups and individuals that appoint hospital board members are: a state governor, a mayor, a city council, a county board, a district board, a bishop, and the ruling body of a religious order.

The advantages of the appointed board are:

- The elected or corporate authority can exercise control over the board and thus over the system and its activities.

- Board members can be appointed according to the criteria and values of the appointing authority.
- Board members can be appointed to advance specific agendas of special concern to the appointing authority.

The disadvantages of the appointed board are:

- The appointing authority may not use a logical method of trustee selection, and thus the board finds that its members lack the needed skills, experience, and knowledge.
- The board is beholden to the appointing authority and is hesitant to make decisions that may be counter to the best interests of the appointing authority, even though they may be in the best interests of the system.
- The board's decision-making process is slowed because the board needs to check all major decisions with the appointing authority before making them.
- Governance responsibility for management oversight and evaluation is often unclear and diffused between the hospital board and the appointing authority.
- The board can exercise no control over dysfunctional members because the power to remove members rests with the appointing authority.
- Self-evaluation tends to be ineffective in improving board performance.

The Self-Perpetuating Board

In the self-perpetuating board, the system board selects its own members, through either an election by the board or board committee, or appointment of new members by the board or board committee. This is the predominant form of governance in, and of new board member selection of, not-for-profit community hospitals and IDSs in the United States.

The advantages of the self-perpetuating board are:

- The board can ensure continuity, stability, and an appropriate mix of member skills, knowledge, and experience through use of specific criteria for new board member selection.
- The board can modify the criteria for selection of new members as circumstances confronting the system change and thus keep the governance function appropriate to changing system needs.
- The board can police itself and remove dysfunctional or nonperforming members to maintain the continuous integrity of board function.

- The board can modify its structure as necessary in a timely manner.
- Self-evaluation is more likely to be effective in maintaining and improving board performance.
- It is the most flexible governance model and the most effective in facilitating fluid, focused, and performance-oriented hospital governance.

The disadvantages of the self-perpetuating board are:

- Without a criteria-based selection process, the board may become too homogeneous in terms of age, gender, professional background, skills, knowledge, and experience.
- The board may be reluctant to enforce performance criteria and remove dysfunctional or nonperforming trustees.
- The board may become insulated from the mission and the community the system is supposed to serve, and thus its decisions may not best serve the system's mission and community.

What Size Should the System Board Be?

Board size often is regarded as a significant structural characteristic that critically affects board function. Often larger boards (those having more than 20 members) are viewed as more likely to be ineffective due to more cumbersome decision-making processes and to diffusion of individual member commitment and involvement. Thus, many governance consultants advocate boards with fewer than 20 members.[3]

However, it is important to remember that board structure does not in itself determine board function; it can only facilitate or inhibit effective board function. Thus, appropriate board size should be determined by each system board's individually defined role and responsibilities. Nevertheless, the trend toward streamlined system boards is evidence of the emerging view that boards with fewer than 20 members tend to be more effective.

The advantages of a board with 20 or more members are:

- Increased ability to represent all segments of the community or the various constituency groups of the health care organization
- The ability to spread the board's work among more members
- The ability to fill a large complement of board committees with board members
- The ability to recruit affluent and politically connected people who will not participate in board functions other than fund-raising and political advocacy

The disadvantages of a board with 20 or more members are:

- A likely ineffectiveness due to more cumbersome decision-making processes
- Diffusion of individual board member commitment and involvement
- The likely development of "cliques" or power being vested in a smaller subgroup of the board
- The tendency to maintain an extensive, laborious board committee structure simply to ensure that all board members can participate on board committees

The advantages of smaller boards (fewer than 10 members) are:

- The potential for faster decision making
- Better focus
- Greater flexibility
- Less communication and coordination effort

The disadvantages of small boards are:

- Burning out board members by spreading them too thin on board and board committee work
- Failing to achieve a good mix of skills, knowledge, and experience on the board
- Unexpected trustee turnover negatively affecting board function due to lack of depth
- The likelihood of one or two individuals exerting disproportionate influence on the board function

Sociopsychological research and theory suggests that the upper limit for effective and efficient group decision making is about 20 individuals. Boards larger than this generate communication and coordination problems, as well as the potential for factions and diffusion of individual trustee responsibility.

A board size of 10 to 20 members is consistent with both effective group process research and the average board size of American not-for-profit IDSs. A board size of 15 or 17 enables a board to be small enough to act as an effective deliberative body and yet large enough to effectively shoulder necessary responsibilities. It also enables a board to function unimpeded by the absence of several trustees from a board meeting. Many governance consultants and researchers recommend a board size of 10 to 20 members.[4]

Should System Board Members Be Compensated?

The issue of board composition leads to another question: Is the notion of volunteer boards appropriate in today's environment? As governance activities become ever more challenging and consume increasing amounts of trustee time, that question can be put another way: Should board members, especially of not-for-profit IDSs, be paid? This issue raises strong feelings because it touches on people's personal views regarding the mission and community purpose of the not-for-profit health care organization, and the need for effective, focused governance of complicated, billion-dollar IDSs.

The advantages of compensating board members are:

- It may make it easier to hold board members accountable for their performance and to expect them to devote more time to board activities.
- It can increase board diversity by encouraging participation from among lower-income members of the community.
- It can attract highly skilled professionals who would otherwise not consider joining the board due to lost income opportunities.
- It can increase attendance at board and committee meetings.

The disadvantages of compensating board members are:

- The community-oriented and charitable mission of the system may be perceived to be diminished.
- It goes against the grain of trusteeship as a civic responsibility.
- It may offend the volunteer trustee's sense of community service.
- It may generate conflicts of interest.
- It may divert board loyalty away from the mission and toward the short-term financial success of the institution because that success may affect their compensation.
- It may make routine board turnover more difficult because members could become reluctant to give up their compensation.
- It may increase board member exposure to director and officer liability because many states grant statutory immunity to volunteer (serving without compensation) directors and officers of not-for-profit corporations.
- It may diminish board utility in the political advocacy arena, where members could be viewed by legislators as "hired guns" or employees of the organization and thus not accorded the same attention and respect as volunteer members of the community.

How Should Physician Involvement in System Governance Be Structured?

According to the American Hospital Association publication *Guidelines: Physician Involvement in Governance of Health Care Institutions*, two types of physician members serve on hospital boards: the physician trustee and the medical staff representative. The publication states that:

> The physician trustee does not serve as a representative of a constituency group, but as an individual who brings to the board important expertise from a particular discipline and whose obligation is to act in the best interest of the institution at all times. On the other hand, a representative of the medical staff to the governing board represents the interests of the institution's medical staff, which, from time to time, may vary from the interests of the institution as a whole.[5]

It goes on to state that physician trustees "should be identified, nominated, elected, or appointed in the same manner as all other board members. Physician Trustees may be selected from among physicians who reside in the community, or in other communities, or from the institution's medical staff."

Mechanisms for physician selection will depend largely on the choices made regarding the first three issues discussed in this chapter. One constraint that should be noted is the Internal Revenue Service (IRS) ruling that prohibits the board of a not-for-profit, tax-exempt health care organization (IRS designation 501[c][3]) from having more than 20 percent of its members be practicing physicians affiliated with the organization.

IDS boards will increasingly find that the hospital medical staff(s) diminishes in importance relative to other physician groups that are specifically designed to link with the hospital and system to manage care and share financial risk. These groups (such as management service organizations [MSOs], physician–hospital organizations [PHOs], physician organizations, and independent practice associations [IPAs]) may be more likely candidates for selection of what used to be known as the "medical staff representative" (perhaps more appropriately designated the "physician group representative").

Should Board Member Terms of Office Be Limited?

The concept of *term limits* as it relates to members of governing boards refers to a limit to the number of years or consecutive terms that a trustee is allowed to serve on a board. As with the issue of board compensation, there has been much debate regarding whether term limits are appropriate in today's changing health care environment.

Currently, most argue that the days of the "lifetime" trustee are gone forever as it is unreasonable to expect volunteer trustees to dedicate significant time and energy and make increasingly critical and far-reaching decisions in these challenging times for indefinite periods. As this view gains currency, there is a trend toward instituting maximum limits on the number of consecutive years that a board member may serve on the board.

The advantages of board member term limits are:

- Boards that do not have regular trustee turnover become stale and complacent.
- It is unreasonable for volunteer trustees to dedicate the significant time and energy required in these challenging times for indefinite periods.
- Board member term limits are necessary to prevent the self-perpetuating board from becoming inbred, as well as to avoid criticism of isolation from the community and key constituency groups.
- It facilitates the review of individual trustee performance at the end of each term (usually three years), and provides the opportunity to adjust the mix of the board and not to reappoint nonperforming trustees.

The disadvantages of board member term limits are:

- Arbitrary limits on the number of terms and tenure expose the board to the risk of losing talented and valuable trustees.
- They prevent continuity in board membership, which in times of massive and rapid changes in health care could be deleterious.

Should the IDS Corporate Parent Be a Not-for-Profit Entity?

In the current health care environment, there is a crosscurrent of thought on the relative merits of traditional not-for-profit health care versus for-profit health care. The current rise of investor-owned hospital companies and managed care organizations, combined with the challenges and pressures experienced by traditional not-for-profit hospitals has fueled this debate. Whether for-profits will gain a lasting position in the American health care market remains to be seen; however, a comparison of the relative advantages and disadvantages of for-profit and not-for-profit structures indicates the significant impact these options can have on system governance.

Not-for-Profit Corporate Entity

The advantages of a not-for-profit corporate entity are:

- Access to tax-exempt bond financing, which provides access to less expensive capital (assuming the entity is a 501[c][3] organization)
- Exemption from certain taxes (again assuming the entity is a 501[c][3] organization)
- Local control of the organization through a community-based, local governance structure
- An organization and governance process that is values based and mission driven

The disadvantages of a not-for-profit corporate entity are:

- Diffusion of governance control because the issue of ownership tends to be unclear
- The potential for less cost efficiency due to the diffusion of purpose often seen in not-for-profits
- IRS regulations restricting the number of physicians on the board to no more than 20 percent
- Increasingly onerous regulations and requirements of the IRS, the Justice Department, and the state attorney general regarding the provision of community benefit to justify tax-exempt status

For-Profit Corporate Entity

The advantages of a for-profit corporate entity are:

- Focused governance through clear identification of the owner and the profit-making purpose of the organization
- No limit on the number of physicians or senior corporate executives who can serve as board members
- Tends to be more successful than not-for-profits in controlling costs and providing cost-efficient care
- Less regulatory and legislative requirements and encumbrances

The disadvantages of a for-profit corporate entity are:

- Focus on profits and organizational viability instead of on achieving a community-based mission

- A blurring of the distinction between governance and management and the resulting consolidation of power in the executive management
- The potential alienation of the community because the organization pursues profitability and possibly merges or sells its assets to another for-profit system
- The potential for no local control of health care delivered in the community

Oakwood Healthcare System: A Case Study in Restructuring

Because it can be mind-numbing to delve into the depths of these issues and options, it is always useful to consider them in relation to the whole. Toward that end, the following case study is provided to show how Oakwood Healthcare System (OHS), headquartered in Dearborn, Michigan, wrestled with these options to create a new governance structure and process.

OHS began an aggressive transition effort in 1995 to become an IDS. At the time, its system characteristics were:

- Six hospitals, including five general acute care facilities and one tertiary facility, with a system total of 2,000 licensed beds
- More than 1,000 affiliated physicians, about one-third of which were primary care physicians
- 21 ambulatory care delivery sites
- A continuing care retirement community with 250 independent and 60 assisted living units and a 200-bed skilled nursing facility
- An additional 200-bed skilled nursing facility
- Two home health agencies
- An interest in an insurance vehicle with health maintenance organization (HMO), preferred provider organization (PPO), and point-of-service product lines

Among the many challenges faced by the chief executive officer (CEO), Jerry Fitzgerald, and the board and physician leadership as they embarked upon this massive change process were physician integration, the redesign of clinical processes, risk-bearing capability, integrated information technology, and restructuring governance. To address these issues in an integrated fashion, OHS created a 22-person transition team composed of system board members, physicians, and administrators. The team's purpose was to oversee and coordinate the activities and recommendations of many specific design teams, one of which was the governance design team.

The governance design team was charged with responsibility for developing recommendations to create a governance structure that would facilitate IDS formation and function and improve the overall governance process and function. The team consisted of the system CEO, four physician leaders, and four members of the system board, and the team was facilitated by an outside consultant with content expertise in governance.

Following the process for governance restructuring described in chapter 5, the team first developed a set of governance principles to guide the redesign process. It then assessed its current governance structure and concluded that it had what amounted to a centralized governance function but a decentralized governance structure.

The system had evolved a decentralized, organizational governance structure on a de facto basis that had resulted in 21 standing boards. This governance structure generated confusion in relative roles and responsibilities among the boards, consumed an inordinate amount of executive management time, and resulted in a cumbersome and redundant decision-making process.

This was viewed as inefficient, likely to cause other problems down the path of integration, and an unacceptable model for effective IDS governance. The team then considered the universe of conceptual governance principles and options and developed the following recommendations to be submitted for approval to the transition team:

- The system would have a modified centralized governance structure with a minimum number of subsidiary boards, with three to four boards suggested.
- The parent board of the system should govern a not-for-profit entity with the potential for-profit subsidiary organizations. The parent board would have ultimate authority and reserved powers for all system components with the exception of certain limited issues where consent would be required from a subsidiary board (such as an MSO board) on a specific issue.
- The subsidiary boards would be organized by function, as opposed to region or organization. The suggested functional distinctions, each with its own board, would be physician entities, insurance, and care delivery.
- The system board would be composed of 15 members, including three physicians—one elected from the primary physician entity (not the medical staffs) and two selected through the normal board member selection process to be established for the system board; the system CEO; one system executive vice-president or medical director; three members chosen from large purchasers of health care; four members from the communities of the system; and three members from health care–related industries and organizations such

as medical schools, pharmaceutical companies, and insurance companies.
- The system board members would be compensated and subject to a term limit of three years, with a maximum limit of three consecutive terms. Once a board member reached the term limit, he or she could be reappointed to the board after a one-year interval. During his or her absence from the board, the member would be eligible to serve on board committees.
- The system board would have a standing governance committee whose duties would include board member recruitment and orientation; oversight and planning of board education and retreats; board self-evaluation; and continuous governance improvement through application of the effective governance pyramid (discussed in chapter 4).
- Where legal or other restrictions require that a specific organization have its own board (such as a home care agency), that board would be an "internal operations" board consisting of a few senior managers and no outside directors.

The transition team unanimously approved the recommendations, and the governance design team began to address development of strategies to implement them, including a plan to structure and compose the new system board. The entire set of governance redesign recommendations was scheduled to be presented to the current OHS board for consideration and approval at its retreat in June 1996.

Conclusion

Framing a set of issues such as those presented in this chapter, and understanding the relative advantages and disadvantages of each, can help clarify and strengthen governance restructuring. However, it is important to remember that no single solution to any of these issues will work equally well for every organization. The best resolution to any issue is that which most accurately reflects the unique needs, culture, and mission of the organization, which effective governance is designed to support.

References

1. Pointer, D. D., and Ewell, C. M. *Really Governing: How Health System and Hospital Boards Can Make More of a Difference.* Albany, NY: Del Mar Publishers Inc., 1994, p. 84.

2. Pointer, D. D., Alexander, J. A., and Zuckerman, H. S. Loosening the gordian knot of governance in integrated health care delivery systems. *Frontiers of Health Services Management* 11(3):20, Spring 1995.
3. Pointer and Ewell, p. 159.
4. Pointer and Ewell.
5. American Hospital Association. *Guidelines: Physician Involvement in Governance of Health Care Institutions.* Chicago: AHA, 1987.

Chapter 7

Conclusion

New mind-sets and structural characteristics are necessary for governance to effectively lead health care into the future. An integrated health care delivery and financing system requires integrated, systems-oriented, mission-based governance. The challenge for boards is to become changemasters not only for their organizations, but also for themselves. In fact, before a board can meaningfully change its organization, it must change itself.

Boards are faced with a series of difficult, interconnected decisions that will do far more than simply determine the survival and future success of their health care organizations and, more important, the fulfillment of their missions. They are confronting issues and decisions that will determine the very existence of mission-based, values-driven health care for American society in the future.

These momentous decisions will include, but are not limited to, issues such as:

- Reducing the overcapacity of a system or health care organization to make it consistent with the demand for ever more efficient services.
- Clearly defining the community and truly serving it. For example, will the system actually serve the entire community or only its own enrolled populations?
- Recognizing that, absent imposed constraints, there is infinite demand for health care services and a finite supply of health care resources. In response, ethically based, consistently applied approaches to rationing health care services will need to be developed, implemented, and communicated to the community.
- Choosing between several strategic directions that are inherently exclusionary to certain physicians or groups of physicians.
- Realizing that it will be impossible to transform a hospital or other health care organization into an integrated delivery system (IDS)

and bring everyone associated with the old organization into the new one. Some employees may lose their jobs, some board members may be displaced, and many physicians may not be able to earn a living practicing within the system.
- Rejecting the hospital paradigm and overcoming the paradox of the hospital funding development of the system that then contributes to the diminution, and possibly dissolution, of the hospital.
- Developing new definitions of health and new measures of health care quality.
- Balancing the need to be increasingly efficient, aggressively competitive, and financially viable, with the preservation and pursuit of the mission.

These and many other monumental issues face the boards of today's health care systems and organizations. However, before a board can begin to meaningfully address such issues, it must be able to control itself. Before a board can control the massive systemic levers that will affect these monumental issues, it must be able to control the levers of effective governance.

What are the levers of effective governance, the variables that a board must control if it is truly to become an effective leader and an agent of controlled, positive change? Simply put, they are:

1. A board must control its single most precious commodity, the time its members spend together.
2. To control this important governance lever, a board must control its agenda.
3. To make its agenda meaningful, a board must control the information it receives.
4. To respond to the information efficiently, a board must control its structures.
5. Once a board has controlled the preceding four levers of effective governance, it can then control the fifth and most important lever: how the board makes meaningful decisions and sets robust policy.

If a board cannot control itself, it will be unable to control the system or organization it putatively governs. To control itself, a board not only must be willing to transform itself in the process of leading its system or organization toward change and integration, but it also must have the discipline to act and the framework to make its action meaningful.

The framework is supplied through tools discussed in this book such as the effective governance pyramid, the structural options for IDS governance, and the process for conducting a governance restructuring project. The discipline, resolve, and will to change must be supplied by each health care organization board itself.

However, the discipline and will to change is a critical piece of transformational governance. Too often, this develops only when a board confronts a crisis. The need to respond to the crisis creates an immediate governance consciousness of the need for change. Although this reactive approach may have had limited success in the past, where more stable and predictable periods were the norm and change was largely incremental, it now is antiquated and dangerous. Today, boards must create the consciousness of change not to *respond* to crises but, rather, to *prevent* them.

Thus, the will and determination to change must be intrinsic, must come from within the board. It comes from the board focusing on the future (as opposed to monitoring the past) and balancing the demands of future trends against the culture, mission, and values of the system. From the dynamic tension created by these two forces (how can we retain the essence of what we are while changing to meet the demands of the future?) comes the motivation for governance transformation.

In his autobiography, Mohandas Gandhi stated: "You must make yourself what you want the world to become."[1] This simple statement has a powerful message for boards of health care organizations:

- If you wish to be an integrated system, you must provide integrated, systems-oriented governance.
- If you wish to restructure your organization for greater efficiency and quality, you must restructure your boards for more effective governance and leadership.
- If your organization must merge, affiliate, or otherwise change to effectively pursue its mission, the board must lead this process through its willingness to change its authority, structure, composition, and function.

Effective health care systems and organizations require effective governance. Now more than ever, the future of the American health care system is in the hands of its leaders—the governing boards.

Reference

1. Gandhi, M. K. *Autobiography: The Story of My Experiments with Truth.* New York City: Dover, 1983, p. 152.

Appendix

Case Examples of Governance in Integrated Delivery Systems

Just as no single model for integrated delivery system (IDS) or network formation can be applied successfully in every community, no one model or approach to governance will work equally well in every situation. As discussed in this book, the best approach to governance is that which functions most effectively to support the individual system's mission and goals.

Several different case examples of IDS governance—Henry Ford Health System in Detroit (spring 1995), Sharp HealthCare in San Diego (winter 1994–1995), and Borgess Health Alliance in Kalamazoo, Michigan (fall 1995)—are presented in this appendix. The dates when each case example was originally prepared are included here to reinforce a critical point about governance restructuring: that effective governance evolves in response to issues and needs facing the organization. The governance function and structure of these organizations has and will continue to change as each integrated system develops. For example, as the partnership between Sharp HealthCare and Columbia/HCA evolves, governance will likely reflect the mission, values, and needs of the emerging organization.

These case examples, therefore, present a snapshot of governance as it continues to evolve. The examples are by no means prescriptive or static. They are included here to provide both ideas and insights from organizations that are undergoing governance restructuring. The case examples are perhaps most striking and useful not for their similarities but for their differences. They indicate a variety of unique approaches being taken by different organizations as they strive to structure governance to meaningfully contribute to system success.

Each case example discusses the history and development of an IDS and the evolution of its approach to governance. The sections address

---

The case examples of IDS governance, written by Mary K. Totten and James E. Orlikoff, are adapted and reprinted, with permission, from The Governance Institute, La Jolla, California.

governance structure and function; board composition, roles, responsibilities, and decision-making authority; communication among and to boards; board member education; and emerging issues and challenges for governance. They also include advice and "lessons learned."

Henry Ford Health System

The Henry Ford Health System (HFHS), a nonprofit directorship corporation serving southeastern Michigan, was established in 1915 when auto pioneer Henry Ford founded Henry Ford Hospital in Detroit. Today, it is a network of health promotion, diagnosis, treatment, research, education, medical equipment, home health, and health care financing services. HFHS includes five hospitals, with an additional four hospitals managed under a joint venture with Mercy Health Services. Thirty-six ambulatory care facilities are part of the system, as well as two nursing homes. HFHS also includes Health Alliance Plan (HAP), Michigan's largest health maintenance organization (HMO) serving more than 3,500 employers and 460,000 members. HAP owns Medical Value Plan, a nonprofit HMO serving 35,500 members and 150 employer groups in Toledo. The Fund for Henry Ford Hospital, also part of HFHS, is an endowment used to fund research.

Almost 2,200 physicians are part of HFHS—1,000 in the Henry Ford Medical Group and approximately 1,200 in private practice. The Henry Ford Health Sciences Center integrates teaching, research, and advanced patient care. The Henry Ford School for Health Sciences offers physician residency programs as well as nursing and allied health education programs. More than 17,000 full- and part-time employees work in HFHS, which is the state's eighth-largest employer.

In 1994, HFHS earned $1.5 billion in revenue. The system provides more than $40 million annually in uncompensated care. Additionally, HFHS is significantly involved in managed care. About 50 percent of its operating revenue comes from capitated contracts.

Development of the current system began in the mid-1970s when HAP affiliated with HFHS. Additional hospitals were added during the 1980s. The system's diverse, broad scope of services supports its mission and vision. (See figure A-1.)

Key characteristics of HFHS include:

- Integration of service delivery and financing, with an emphasis on managed care
- Employed medical groups and an extensive ambulatory care network
- Diversified services spanning the continuum of care
- A commitment to education and research

Figure A-1. Henry Ford Health System Mission and Vision Statements

Mission

Henry Ford Health System is a national leader in health care. Our essential priority is to provide exceptional quality, cost-effective care, strengthened by excellence in education and research. We work together to improve health and the quality of life in the communities of southeastern Michigan and the neighboring regions.

Vision

We are expanding the health care delivery system concept through our pioneering vision and leadership's commitment to innovation, always striving to improve access, cost-effectiveness, and quality of care:

- We are designing our services and programs around the needs of our patients and the communities we serve.
- We are integrating our services to provide complete, lifelong health care in ways our customers find easy to use.
- We are enhancing the value of our services through innovative partnerships, managed care, and health education programs.
- To continually improve our services, we measure patient satisfaction and community health.

Governance at Henry Ford Health System

Governance structure and function at HFHS has evolved with the system. HFHS is governed by a system board and is the sole member or shareholder, with specific reserved powers, of all its affiliated entities. Currently, HFHS has 19 governing boards involving more than 200 volunteer community leaders. Each separate legal entity in the system is governed by a board; operating divisions have boards that act in an advisory, community relations capacity.

Board Structure and Composition

The system board has 42 elected or ex officio members, including the chairs of all subsidiary boards; additional representation from HAP; up to four physician trustees, including the chief medical officer (CMO) and the system chief executive officer (CEO). The size of subsidiary boards varies, with most having 15 community members. The smallest is the three-member SHA Realty Board.

Membership overlaps among many HFHS boards. In addition to designated membership for subsidiary board chairs on the system board, other boards that do not have designated members rotate their representatives to the system board. The board of The Fund for Henry Ford Hospital is elected annually and has the same members as the executive committee of the system board.

The system board meets three times a year and has an active committee structure. The executive committee acts for the full board between board meetings. The parent board has the following standing committees: executive, chairman's council, compensation, finance, human resources, nominating, philanthropy, and quality. The system board also makes liberal use of ad hoc committees when needed.

Board Roles and Responsibilities

HFHS is consolidating its corporate structure, which will streamline and centralize its governance and create new board models and roles. The system board retains duties such as:

- Article and bylaws amendments
- Budget and debt approval
- Strategic planning
- Appointment of all trustees and board chairs
- Oversight of system quality
- Philanthropy

The system is regionalizing its operations and merging acute care and ambulatory physician functions within a region under a single advisory board. The primary role of these regional boards is oversight of quality and customer relations. Specific regional board powers include:

- Oversight of all regional activities
- Promoting coordination across the system
- With the system board, selection and evaluation of the regional CEO and CMO
- Participation in plan and budget development
- Monitoring plans and budgets
- Monitoring quality and patient satisfaction
- Joint Commission on Accreditation of Healthcare Organizations' governing body functions, including credentialing
- Maintaining positive relations with private medical staff
- Advocacy
- Nomination and orientation of new trustees
- Board evaluation
- Communication of community needs and system needs, plans and issues

Regional board membership typically includes the CEO and the CMO for the region; representation from the HMO; additional physician representation, such as a hospital chief of staff; and community representatives.

The committee structure for these boards is developing, but usually includes quality, finance, and nominating committees. Because regional boards are advisory, their committees can include nontrustee members.

Although some boards have members who act in a more representative capacity, such as the chief of staff of a hospital, HFHS stresses a broader role for all of its trustees. The system looks for trustees who are big-picture thinkers in touch with community needs.

In general, board meeting frequency varies by organization.

All trustee terms are three years long. A maximum of three consecutive three-year terms, with one year off, is becoming the standard at HFHS. Some advisory boards still have a two-term limit.

Communication, Education, and Development

HFHS uses a variety of approaches to maintain and build awareness of issues and overall system operation among its board members. In addition to overlapping membership among boards, meetings, publications, and education programs are available to HFHS board members.

The chairmen's council, composed of all-volunteer board chairs, meets quarterly. The council is responsible for nominating and orienting new trustees to the system, as well as dealing with issues of concern to all HFHS boards, such as policy review and standardization of trustee terms. Information exchange is promoted through system reports, which include activities and issues from each organization that affect the entire system. An agenda planning meeting is held with the system CEO and those who staff HFHS boards to prepare for the chairmen's council and discuss topics such as nominating information. These agenda planning sessions facilitate how to further standardize and integrate HFHS board function.

The more than 200 trustee community leaders who participate in HFHS governance meet annually with management and medical staff leadership for a half-day caucus that provides opportunities for education and socializing, and promotes integration. The caucus usually includes an address from the system CEO, an outside speaker, an interactive exercise, and a final full-group session.

Every other week, HFHS President and CEO Gail L. Warden writes *CEO Briefings,* a newsletter for all board members. It includes information about key system board activities; awards and honors received by those in the system; announcements; an overview of national issues, such as health reform; articles about important health care issues; and a meeting calendar.

A systemwide orientation is held every March for new HFHS trustees and is supplemented with additional orientation sessions held by local boards.

Education for trustees is typically accomplished within the system; it is not customary to send board members to outside educational meetings.

HFHS has staff dedicated to supporting its boards. The corporate vice-president and secretary is devoted full-time to board support and has four designated assistants. Together, they staff all parent board and committee meetings and the board meetings of most HFHS subsidiaries, totaling 75 meetings per year. An additional 75 meetings are staffed by the key management liaison and staff for the remaining boards.

An officers committee, composed of the chair and three vice-chairs of the system board, also meets informally as needed with the system CEO to discuss emerging issues.

Emerging Governance Issues

"In an era when the health care industry is downsizing, many conclude that integrated systems should downsize their governance structures. I believe that HFHS is enhanced by having trustees who represent a variety of perspectives and communities. Our broad base increases involvement, creates opportunities to develop better community leaders, and enhances integration in ways that would not be possible if we had one 15-member board governing the entire enterprise. The real question is whether a system wishes to maintain its community base," said Gail L. Warden, president and CEO.

As HFHS continues to evolve, new issues are confronting the system and its trustees.

According to Corporate Vice-President and Secretary Anita Fennessey Watson, although HFHS boards contribute overall to the success of the system, improvements are continuing to be made in how work is assigned to various boards.

"By 1997, we will have fully implemented trustee term limits and will have right-sized our boards, allowing us to comprehensively address issues such as leadership succession planning," Watson explained. "Our regionalization process also is helping us crystallize the role and function of our boards so that we have the right boards, with the right leaders addressing the right issues in a timely manner, thereby enhancing the overall value of governance in the system."

Sometimes boards of newly acquired HFHS organizations continue to operate, for a time, in their traditional way, Watson added, and it could be beneficial for them to assimilate more quickly into the HFHS governance structure and function.

Some experts feel that board compensation will become more common as systems emerge and more is asked of the board members that govern them. HFHS does not compensate its board members at this time and feels most trustees view their HFHS board work as community service and therefore do not view compensation to be appropriate.

Keys to Success

In evaluating the development of its governance structure and function, HFHS has identified several factors that contribute to success:

- Board members who understand their strong leadership and policy-making role
- Several avenues for communication among boards and key leaders
- Good working relationships among board members, management, and support staff
- The vision of the system's CEO
- Ongoing, regular communication among the system CEO, board chairs, and officers
- Education about emerging health care issues
- Extensive system board and CEO evaluation processes
- A centrally coordinated function for governance that helps integrate boards systemwide

"With 200 volunteers participating in our governance process, we need central coordination to operate smoothly and effectively," Watson said. "A professionally driven governance function also elevates the importance of boards within the system."

In setting up a governance structure for an IDS, Watson advised that the process be led by the board. "Use consultants wisely to achieve change," she said.

Watson also encouraged newly forming systems to make the tough decisions about what stays and what goes, when combining organizations, to get more value out of what is established. "It's a new world," she said, "and systems operate very differently from the acute care hospitals we were used to governing."

Figure A-2 summarizes the main features of the governance function at HFHS.

Sharp HealthCare

Sharp HealthCare, a not-for-profit public benefit corporation serving the San Diego region, began as a single hospital named in memory

Figure A-2. Henry Ford Health System: Governance at a Glance

Total number of boards: 19

Total number of volunteer trustees: More than 200

Board composition: Community representatives, physicians, and management

Board committees: 8 of parent board

Board function: Oversight of system mission, quality, customer relations, and community needs

Board meeting frequency: System board, 3 times/year; most others quarterly

Board terms: A maximum of three consecutive three-year terms

Guiding principles of governance: Centralized decision making, central coordination of and support for boards, emphasis on meeting customer and community needs

---

of Donald N. Sharp of San Diego. Today, it is a network of six acute care hospitals, four skilled nursing centers, more than 15 ambulatory care clinics, and an array of specialized services, including home health, outpatient surgery, sports medicine, and postsurgical recovery. Sharp also offers San Diego employers an insurance program that covers health, wellness, and occupational medicine for employees and their families.

More than 2,200 primary and specialty care physicians are on the medical staffs of one or more of the six Sharp hospitals. Sharp also has developed a three-year Family Practice Residency Program, which is expected to begin accepting residents this fall. Just over 10,000 employees work throughout the Sharp system.

Sharp HealthCare is predominantly involved in managed care. Six medical groups that accept prepaid health plans are affiliated with Sharp HealthCare. Sharp Health Plan is the system's not-for-profit HMO. Sharp HealthCare covers a population of approximately 900,000, which includes some 300,000 capitated lives and an estimated 600,000 managed care lives.

Development of the Sharp system began in 1986 to ensure that Sharp would be able to continue to fulfill its mission (shown in figure A-3) and compete with competitors such as the Kaiser Permanente system. Key characteristics of the Sharp system include:

- An emphasis on physician groups
- Hospitals strategically located throughout Sharp's service area
- A centralized management structure
- Coordinated clinical and management operations

Figure A-3. Sharp HealthCare Mission Statement

> The mission of Sharp is to improve the health of those we serve with a commitment to excellence in all that we do. Our goal is to offer quality care and services that set community standards, exceed patients' expectations, and are provided in a caring, convenient, cost-effective, and accessible manner.

Sharp strives to maintain a balance among health care providers at all levels of the system. Physicians, executives, and professionals are represented in management teams throughout Sharp HealthCare. Medical groups and institutions share risk and are represented in decision making as the system grows and develops.

Governance at Sharp HealthCare

Although a governance structure for Sharp HealthCare was designed prior to formation of the system, governance, like Sharp HealthCare itself, has continued to evolve. For example, twice since 1988, governance of the system has been revisited, with the most recent change being the addition of more medical group representation on the parent board.

Sharp has a parent board, the San Diego Hospital Association Board of Directors; five boards to oversee the hospitals; three fundraising boards; three clinic boards; a for-profit corporation board; and a health plan board. A community board, made up of representatives of the boards of each Sharp organization, meets in conjunction with the San Diego Hospital Association Board. The community board provides a forum for board members to learn about local and national health care issues, and allows board members to review and comment on Sharp's activities and give advice on policies and procedures. The community board is charged with bringing a community perspective to Sharp's activities and is viewed as a place to recruit new volunteer participants for the Sharp system.

Board Structure and Composition

The parent board has 17 members, including seven physicians from the hospitals and medical groups and the CEO, who serves ex officio with vote. The size of subsidiary boards varies, with 5 members on the board of the for-profit subsidiary, 7 members on medical group boards, 15 members on most hospital boards, and 38 members on the system foundation board. Overall, Sharp HealthCare has some 180 board members.

Sharp strives to maintain a balance of community, hospital, medical group, and management representation on its boards. Each board has a combination of representative and at-large members.

Membership overlaps among many Sharp boards. The parent board and its executive committee include members from subsidiary boards. Membership overlaps between the foundation and hospital boards, the clinic and foundation boards, and the clinic and hospital boards.

Board membership did not rotate until recently, because leadership continuity during system formation was considered essential. Four years ago, Sharp adopted a rotating model of governance as the size and scope of the system increased.

The number of board committees is kept to a minimum. The parent board has the following committees:

- Audit
- Nominating and bylaws
- Finance
- Executive
- Community care
- Institutional care

The executive committee has 11 members, including the chair of the parent board, the CEO of Sharp HealthCare, two representatives from the Institutional Care Committee, two representatives from the Community Care Committee, and five at-large members. This committee oversees the operating entities.

The Institutional Care Committee has 11 members, including five physicians, the four chairs of the hospital boards, and two management representatives. This committee is not a decision-making body, but discusses how new programs and services at each hospital will affect the entire system.

The Community Care Committee also has 11 members, including the chairs of three corporate subsidiaries, six physicians, the executive vice-president for community care, and the CEO of Sharp HealthCare. This committee functions in the same manner as the Institutional Care Committee, but focuses on activities at the medical groups and specialized facilities.

Subsidiary boards generally have few committees and act primarily in an advisory capacity.

Board Roles and Responsibilities

Roles and responsibilities vary between parent and subsidiary boards. The parent board is responsible for:

- Setting direction and policy for the system
- Reviewing and approving new business
- Approving budget and capital expenditures
- Reviewing and approving the consent agendas of all subsidiary boards

The operating boards are responsible for:

- The quality and service of their respective organizations, which is evaluated using a variety of corporate data
- Monitoring financial performance against budget
- Providing input from the community

In addition, the governing board of each hospital is responsible for final decision making on medical staff issues, such as credentialing, which are handled directly by the full board. Foundation boards also are responsible for fund-raising issues.

Although some board members, such as hospital chiefs of staff, represent medical staff issues and concerns at the board level, they also are expected to play the same role as all other board members—to be big-picture thinkers and provide broad oversight for their organization. Parent board members also are required to play a system role.

Board Function

Overall, governance at Sharp is both centralized and decentralized. Day-to-day operations are decentralized, but areas such as finance are handled at the system board level.

Sharp's parent board functions like a corporate board in that it plays more of an oversight role rather than initiating activities. Its primary responsibility is to monitor and evaluate management ideas and proposals, and ensure that new initiatives are financially feasible and consistent with Sharp's mission. The parent board spends the majority of its time reviewing strategic direction, new programs, and new markets; evaluating financial performance; and monitoring quality across the system.

Sharp's subsidiary board members are expected to maintain a community focus, rather than manage their institutions. Sharp strives to represent local customers and constituencies on its boards and expects board members to be in touch with community needs, as well as oversee service quality and financial performance.

Sharp's boards function to support an overall goal of completing the decision-making cycle within 30 days—from management review and recommendation through final approval by the parent board. Boards meet in sequence, within the third week and first two days of the fourth week of the month, to accomplish this goal.

In general, board meeting frequency varies by organization. Hospital and medical group boards meet monthly or bimonthly, and the community and San Diego Hospital Association boards meet together quarterly.

Communication, Education, and Development

Sharp uses a variety of approaches to maintain and build awareness of its overall operation among its board members. In addition to overlapping membership among boards, several publications and education programs are available to Sharp board members.

Two publications, *Sharp Today,* a bimonthly newsletter, and *Health,* a quarterly health and wellness magazine, are sent to board members. *Sharp Points,* a briefing from the system CEO, is sent as needed. *Board Briefs* is a newsletter prepared individually for subsidiary boards. Pertinent news articles also are sent to board members. The system CEO keeps in regular contact with system board members and meets with the board chair at least twice a week.

A formal orientation is conducted for all board members. Every board member is oriented to the system and, in more detail, to their individual organization. The system CEO and the board chair conduct the orientation for parent board members; subsidiary board members are oriented by their chief executive, board chair, and one other board member. Orientation is continued throughout the year at board meetings. Sharp management attends these meetings and tailors education toward specific needs of individual boards.

Because the Sharp system has 180 board members, the cost of board education is an issue. Education is conducted locally and directed primarily to hospital board members through quarterly meetings and additional meetings as needed. Topics have included health care reform, integration of clinical systems, development of Sharp's information system, and community projects.

No single employee at any level in the system is devoted to supporting Sharp's boards; this is seen as the responsibility of the top executive at each organization in the system.

Emerging Governance Issues

Sharp believes that system governance will continue to evolve as the system itself evolves. According to Sharp HealthCare CEO Peter Ellsworth, "It's easy to say that over time we will decrease the number of our governing boards, but I'm not sure that this would be the best approach."

Overall, Sharp believes in small-sized boards and leadership continuity. However, one issue facing Sharp is how to continue gaining representation from the various constituencies served by the system while maintaining continuity and excellence among its board members. Like many organizations, Sharp is challenged to retain its valued board members and at the same time identify and bring onto its boards new leaders who will bring fresh perspectives and skills.

"Because we have a number of boards, we have an opportunity to evaluate our current board talent and appoint them to board or ad hoc committees to maintain their interest and help them move up through the leadership structure," Ellsworth said.

Some experts feel that board compensation will become more common as systems emerge and more is asked of the board members who govern them. Sharp does not compensate its board members at this time and feels most would view compensation negatively.

Keys to Success

In evaluating development of its governance structure and function, Sharp has identified several factors that contribute to success:

- System leaders need to establish a clear definition of roles and responsibilities between and among boards.
- Because systems are large and complex, boards should take a corporate approach to governance, focusing on maintaining the mission rather than hands-on involvement.
- Because the process of building an integrated system is complicated and takes time, leadership continuity is essential.
- Board members need to be courageous—willing and able to make tough decisions and take responsibility for them.
- Board members must be committed, able to understand, and buy in to what the system is trying to accomplish. Being on the board should be high on each member's personal priority list. Members need to be able to devote their time and stand by, if needed.

"The governance model we're evolving makes a lot of sense," Ellsworth said, "but we found that you can't try to change the world on the first day. The goal is to evolve the thinking of your system's boards so that they can deal with problems facing the system as it develops."

Figure A-4 summarizes the main features of the governance function at Sharp HealthCare.

Borgess Health Alliance

This case example profiles governance at Borgess Health Alliance (BHA), an integrated health care system serving southwestern Michigan. BHA is sponsored by the Sisters of St. Joseph of Nazareth, Michigan, and is a member of the Sisters of St. Joseph Health System, Inc.

BHA owns two hospitals, including its flagship, Borgess Medical Center; two nursing homes; an ambulatory care corporation; a preferred provider organization and third-party administrative service; and a medical foundation, which was formed with a group of primary care physicians. Four additional hospitals are affiliated with the Alliance, with plans currently under way to merge one of these hospitals with Borgess Medical Center. BHA participates in joint ventures and other collaborative arrangements to operate and/or provide a broad range of services, including an HMO in an affiliation with Blue Cross/Blue Shield of Michigan; other insurance products; mobile imaging services; ground and air transport; an outpatient cancer treatment center; home health and durable medical equipment services; and graduate medical education.

A primary focus for BHA is to capture a greater share of the emerging managed care/capitated marketplace.

"A few years ago, we began to look at what was happening across the country," said R. Timothy Stack, BHA president and CEO. "It was becoming clear that physicians and hospitals needed to be integrated financially and organizationally. We studied integrated health care systems across the country to determine what made them "systems" and, through our Borgess Institute for Health Care Leadership, began to educate our board, medical staff, management, and subsidiaries so we could proceed

Figure A-4. Sharp HealthCare: Governance at a Glance

Total number of boards: 1 community board, 1 parent board, 13 subsidiary boards

Total number of board members: 180

Board composition: Management, hospital, and medical group physicians, community representatives

Board committees: 6 of parent board

Board function: Oversight of management ideas and proposals, new programs and services, finances and service quality; emphasis on community needs and system mission

Board meeting frequency: Varies by organization, either monthly, bimonthly, or quarterly

Board terms: Varies among boards, either one-, two-, or three-year terms

Guiding principles of governance: Small-sized boards; leadership continuity; expeditious decision making; oversight, not management with a common knowledge base. We felt that integration of both service delivery and financing was essential," Stack said. "We focused first on integration with physicians and are now moving further into the insurance and financing aspects of system development."

Managed care penetration in southwest Michigan is low, but increasing, Stack said. Over the past three years, a coalition of Kalamazoo-area employers has helped to organize managed care in the area and currently represents approximately 60,000 lives. BHA's total service area includes nine to ten counties, with a population of about 900,000.

"Because we're in a first-generation managed care market, our challenge is to create a future-oriented system in a market that isn't there yet," Stack said. This challenge is embodied in BHA's mission, vision, and reorganization goals. (See figure A-5.)

Governance at Borgess Health Alliance

After the strategic plan for the delivery and financing system was in place, system governance and then management were reorganized. "We restructured in that order because our educational process showed us we needed to first determine what kind of organization we wanted to be,"

Figure A-5. Borgess Health Alliance Mission, Vision, and Reorganization Goals

Mission

The mission of Borgess Health Alliance is to provide an integrated health system, directly or through collaboration, that will be clinically and fiscally accountable for improving the health status of southwest Michigan.

Vision

Evolve Borgess Health Alliance into an integrated network with the capability to manage capitated lives by controlling and integrating both a health care delivery system and a health care financing system that serves residents of southwestern Michigan.

Reorganization Goals

- Transition from a medical center into a regional integrated delivery system
- Develop and implement a physician organization
- Develop and implement an integrated financing system (managed care/capitated lives)

Stack said. "The change for us and our board was relatively easy. As far back as 1992, integration, regionalization, and networks were topics of discussion, so the formation of BHA was a natural progression. We have an open-minded, educated board, so it was not a hard push to change.

"Our education efforts really paid off with our board members," he added, "because they were able to see how a medical center board that had existed for more than 100 years needed to relinquish its power and position to the BHA board. Although Borgess Medical Center is still a very significant part of the Alliance, the system is now the primary focus."

Governance at BHA was restructured based on the following assumptions:

- Position BHA to continue to be responsive to health reform, managed care, and a capitated marketplace.
- Restructure governance in keeping with mission, vision, and goals (combine BHA and Borgess Medical Center boards and create subsidiary boards).
- Reduce duplication of effort and maximize utilization of trustee time and interests.
- Provide opportunities to engage additional community representatives to contribute to the governance of BHA.
- Provide opportunities for physician representation in BHA governance.
- Reduce duplication of effort of senior management officers.

BHA's governance structure is a tremendously streamlined version of what used to exist. "Eight years ago, we had more than 30 organizations and 165 board meetings annually," Stack explained. "We've structured BHA governance to reduce time spent for boards and management and to align closely with our vision. For example, we no longer have a separate medical center board because we want our trustees to look beyond individual units to the system as a whole."

The BHA governance structure includes five boards—the BHA board and four others that govern the majority of BHA's activities.

Board Structure and Composition

The 26-member BHA board of trustees provides overall guidance for the system. The majority of BHA board members are members of subsidiary boards; the BHA president and CEO serves with vote. Physicians comprise 15 percent of the BHA Board; two physician trustees represent medical staff issues and the others act as community representatives. The BHA board also includes five members of the Sisters of St. Joseph.

The Borgess Ambulatory Care Corporation board has nine members. It oversees off-site outpatient care and other outreach programs. The Borgess Foundation board oversees not-for-profit fund-raising and charitable activities. It has nine members. ProMed Healthcare is a nonprofit medical foundation that integrates services with those provided by a select group of primary care physicians to enable joint contracting with employers and payers for a full array of health care services. The ProMed board currently has 15 members, 20 percent of whom are primary care physicians. The 15-member Service Delivery and Financing board oversees the medical center, nursing homes, and other aspects of the continuum of care, as well as BHA's managed care activities.

Most BHA boards meet four or five times a year. The ProMed board meets more frequently, on a monthly or bimonthly basis.

The BHA board currently has four committees:

- Executive
- Finance/audit
- Strategic planning
- Board development

The BHA executive committee meets eight to nine times a year and has a compensation subcommittee.

The Service Delivery and Financing board has three committees: executive, joint conference, and services and quality improvement.

Board Role and Function

BHA is a member of the Sisters of St. Joseph Health System and ultimately is accountable to the system board. The chair of the BHA board serves on the health system board. "BHA has a great deal of latitude locally," Stack said.

BHA is developing a model of governance decision making that is both centralized and decentralized.

"We feel that the Alliance is best served by empowered boards," Stack said. "For example, strategic planning for the system is done at the BHA board; however, subsidiary boards then develop their own plans that fit into the overall system plan. Decisions such as physician credentialing are made by the Service Delivery and Financing board. Ultimately, we want decision making to occur at the lowest possible level."

Communication, Education, and Development

BHA uses a variety of methods to communicate with its board members, who receive direct communication on a regular basis and all publications produced by BHA. "We use a variety of approaches because we believe that our boards should hear things first," Stack said. "I also have a tremendously talented group of senior staff who all have access to our boards," he added. BHA does not have a single person responsible for board support, but spreads the responsibility among several senior executives.

BHA provides an orientation to new board members, which focuses on an overview of the Alliance as well as health care industry issues and trends. An annual education retreat for members of all Borgess boards, plus additional management and physicians as well as other education programs, is conducted by the Borgess Institute for Health Care Leadership.

Emerging Governance Issues

Because BHA is a new system, it is working through several issues. "Although our boards are definitely community minded, we are still in a learning curve in terms of thinking and acting like a system," Stack said. "Our board members understand why we are a system, but they are still learning how to govern from a system perspective."

"One of our biggest challenges is that the majority of our revenue still comes from inpatient hospital care," Stack added. "However, we recognize that this will definitely not be the case in the future."

Shifting focus carries with it conflicts that have to be overcome. "We are not really dealing with capitation now in our market, but as we position ourselves to accept it, we encounter conflicting goals," Stack explained. "It's a big challenge to maintain our healthy bottom line and move into managed care and capitated markets where the goal is to maximize the number of covered lives. That's why we combined service delivery and financing under one umbrella so that both sides would need to cooperate and work together."

Stack also said that BHA is learning to walk before it runs. "We initially focused ProMed on integration with primary care physicians," he said, "but now we are concurrently working with specialists who came to us and asked for a role. Together, we can troubleshoot issues and think through solutions as a team."

As the scope of governance expands through system formation, many organizations consider compensating their boards. When BHA asked their board members if they wanted to be compensated, they indicated that compensation would not be appropriate. "Compensation would not be indicative of the value our board members bring to us," Stack said. "We could not compensate them enough. However, the day is coming when board members should be compensated for the time and commitment we ask of them."

Keys to Success

"Although many organizations across the country are still having trouble integrating service delivery and financing, integration of these is critical to a system's success," Stack observed.

"Educating your boards, physicians, employees, and the community before you undertake system formation is very important," he said. "An organization must first educate its key stakeholders and then continue to do so as the system evolves."

Figure A-6 summarizes the main features of the governance function at BHA.

Figure A-6. Borgess Health Alliance: Governance at a Glance

Total number of boards: 1 parent board, 4 subsidiary boards

Total number of current board seats: 74

Board composition: Community representatives, physicians, management, sponsor representatives

Board function: Oversight of system mission, values, and strategic direction; decision making at lowest possible level

Board meeting frequency: Typically four to five times a year

Board terms: Three-year terms

Guiding principles of governance: Streamlined board structure to avoid duplication and ensure best use of board member and staff time; empowered boards; focus on marketplace and community needs

Additional Books of Interest

Strategic Planning in Health Care: A Guide for Board Members

by Ellen F. Goldman and Kevin C. Nolan of Ernst & Young LLP with a finance primer by Jonathan G. Weaver

This book gives board members an overview of the organizational planning process and outlines their specific roles and responsibilities. It also provides details on the tools used for financial oversight as the institution executes its strategic plan. In addition, the book:

- Helps boards of health care organizations better understand the strategic planning process, formulate an organizational vision, and develop effective strategies
- Introduces strategic thinking in the context of current business challenges, such as network development, hospital-physician integration, and the growth of managed care
- Provides direction on reading financial statements, important ratios, and debt capacity calculations

Catalog No. F4-196130 (must be included when ordering)
1994. 140 pages, 12 figures, 6 tables, appendix, glossary, bibliography.
$35.00 (AHA members, $28.00)

Transformational Leadership: Renewing Fundamental Values and Achieving New Relationships in Health Care

by Mary K. Kohles, RN, MSW, William G. Baker, Jr., MD, and Barbara A. Donaho, RN, MA

This book carefully looks at your role as a leader in transforming your organization to meet the challenge of providing compassionate, effective care within the restraints of current and future economic environments. You'll explore the visioning process, the continuous value improvement strategy, interactive planning methods, and the human and system factors that challenge transformational leaders. The book also describes the characteristics of organizations and their leaders that have made successful transformations possible.

Catalog No. F4-001116 (must be included when ordering)
1995. 294 pages, 14 figures, 1 table, 3 appendixes.
$40.00 (AHA members, $32.00)

To order, call TOLL FREE 800-AHA-2626